Autoimmune Cases – Naturally!

Autoimmune Cases – Naturally!

===========================

Treating Autoimmune Disorders Using

Energy Psychology & Naturopathy

Anne Merkel, Ph.D., CNHP

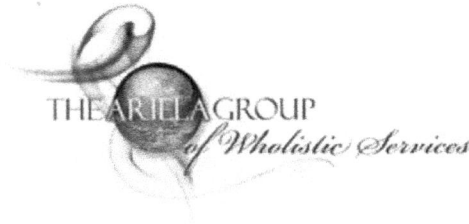

THE ARIELA GROUP
of Wholistic Services

Ariela Group Publications / Mineral Bluff, GA

ISBN: 978-0-9961262-6-7

Library of Congress Control Number: 2015914199
　　　Ariela Group Publications, Mineral Bluff, GA

BISAC: Health & Fitness / General

Join me at these locations to learn more about my Energy Therapy Programs, Services, and Products for Individuals – and - Health & Wellness Practitioners!

For Individuals:

- Body – Mind- Spirit Coaching Services for Individuals:
  www.ArielaGroup.com
- Coaching to use N-hanced EFT & Energy Therapy:
  www.MyEFTCoach.com
- Energy Psychology, Naturopathy, Energy Medicine:
  www.AlchemistAnne.com
- Autoimmune Coaching & Energy Therapy Support FREE Series:
  www.myeftcoach.com/autoimmune-coaching-support-group
- Bonus EFT & Energy Therapy Tapping FREE Series:
  www.arielagroup.com/blog/eft-tapping-group

For Practitioners:

- EFT & Energy Therapy Programs & Packages for Practitioners:
  www.AnneMerkel.com
- EFT & Energy Therapy Mastermind for Practitioners Series:
  www.annemerkel.com/practitioner-mastermind
- Certified Energy Therapy Practitioner Program:
  www.annemerkel.com/energy-therapy-certification
- Books on Amazon by Anne Merkel for Practitioners:
  http://is.gd/AnnesBooks

Autoimmune Information:

- Programs, Interviews, Presentations, Research:
  http://annemerkel.com/autoimmune-programs/

Preface & Acknowledgements

This book could not have been possible without the extensive parade of teachers that have traveled along my path with me. It has taken several professions and lots of life experience for me to be able to bring this book to you. I also wish to thank my many wonderful clients who have presented to my practice with serious issues that they invited me to address. We have learned together about the wondrous powers of the body!

I have included here unique cases with both classic and not-so-normal issue involvement so that you, the reader, may get an idea of the far-reaching scope of issues involved in autoimmune disorders. You may witness my use of a several-step protocol that will be outlined and discussed in more detail in another book. Since each person and each case is so unique, you will notice a difference in how I manage each session and individual.

There are many ways to address autoimmune disorders, and my own is through the emotional component that I find attached to the cases with which I work. There are many tools used in Energy Psychology that can be applied in these autoimmune cases, and you will see evidence here of this. I've also included information from a Naturopathic approach, although the more far-reaching scope of utilizing homeopathy, flower essences, essential oils, and more will be covered elsewhere.

I'd like to specifically thank the following for giving me permission to use their names (or pseudonyms *) in my work with you and other clients: Gerry*, Tanya, Sally, Amanda, Veronica, Helen*, and Kristen.

And, if you suffer from autoimmune, I hope that this book gives you hope and trust that you will NOT need to endure a "life sentence" of suffering!

August, 2015

Contents

Introduction

Hello. I am Anne Merkel, and I am a survivor of autoimmune disorders. I practice as an Energy Psychologist, using various energy therapy tools to help unblock bodies, minds, spirits of stuck energy and emotions, and I specialize in supporting clients who are suffering from autoimmune disorders.

Please allow me to share my own case with you as well as more background information about autoimmune disorders and their possible causes, or at least the causes that I help to clear so that the bodies of my clients can begin to re-balance and return to health.

Realize that any kind of "total" healing must be done via consideration of the "whole" system. So, as I approach each case in a "wholistic" manner I now incorporate what I've learned in 31+ years of post-doctorate study and application. "My toolbox" includes techniques taken from various modalities of energy therapy, energy medicine, and naturopathy. You will notice my advice and application with clients jumps around among my many tools, and I never plan ahead what each client will need in the NOW of a session.

My Story

I was raised in a very conservative Louisville, Kentucky environment by parents who still don't believe in alternative holistic approaches to health. Growing up my body was healthy and athletic. I lived life to the fullest and was only held back by a fall from my horse at age 17.

I was always a good student and talented musician, and found that I was sensitive to the needs of others. My undergraduate majors were music and Spanish with minors in psychology and business. My Masters courses covered international studies, comparative education, applied linguistics, Latin American studies, business, and teaching English as a second or foreign language.

I worked through my graduate school stresses by beating tennis balls around the courts with friends. I'll never forget the day that after a good tennis match with a friend, I took a shower and bent over and four days later I still couldn't stand up. My friend then insisted that he get me some help so he gently threw me in the back of his car and took me to his chiropractor. That was my first introduction to a holistic practitioner. One adjustment and I was pain free. Years before that when I'd fallen off my horse an orthopedist had told me: "You've got to wear a back brace the rest of your life. You'll never be athletic again. Forget about having kids. Pregnancy will be horrible for you." These were nasty words for a teenager's ears. Now this chiropractor said: "You don't have to live with that life sentence of suffering."

I hear about this same "life sentence of suffering" from autoimmune sufferers all of the time. They've been given not a "death sentence" but a "life sentence" of suffering. "Just go home and live with it. It's all in your head. Go home and live with the pain. Get into pain management because you're going to live with the pain the rest of your life. You're going to have to be on these drugs the rest of your life," is what they are often told.

I don't believe any of it because I have always had deep faith in the power of my body. I got up off the ground from the horse accident and I only wear my back brace when I'm skiing black diamonds in Aspen and I know I'm going to land in a pile at the bottom of the mountain,... and I haven't done that for a while.

After this first visit to the chiropractor I was sold! He opened a whole new world to me and I haven't looked back a single time. Years later I even married a chiropractor, and that is when I began to study and apply holistic tools in my own work.

My PhD from Indiana University is in cognitive learning, socio- / psycho-linguistics, how the brain learns and how to best educate and communicate with it. I had been a focused musician for 20 years and then I worked part-time as an academician for 20 years, teaching in 20 colleges and universities, including four MBA programs. At that same time I was in corporate America as a top-level manager, first woman director for one of the biggest companies of a multinational conglomerate. I've always been a Type A personality and over-achiever as well as a Highly Sensitive artist. Both of these profiles are prone to develop autoimmune disorders, as I will point out later.

I married my former husband when he was in chiropractic school, and learned all of the in's and out's of that profession as I was used as a "guinea pig" for the years of clinical application. My husband turned out to be an excellent healer but horrible businessman. I financially supported him for the duration of our seventeen year partnership and we remain friends to this day.

When I was in my early 40s, there came a year when I was totally exhausted all the time. Then I started losing my memory. I couldn't remember details. At first it was just little stuff. I was doing major corporate work, training in front of audiences. I had moments of: "Wait a minute, what am I doing here?" Then my body started hurting very badly with pain all the time. Being a Type A personality, I wouldn't let myself take a nap. "Naps are for lazy people," is what my parents had taught me. But when you get to the point where you're going to die or take a nap, you learn to take naps. Pretty soon I was to the point where I was spending most of my time in bed. I think that particular year I only earned about $6,000 because I couldn't work. I couldn't stand in front of audiences. I couldn't get it together. It was becoming a desperate situation for me and my husband was forced to support me.

After a full year of suffering from Chronic Fatigue Syndrome and Fibromyalgia, one day I screamed at the Universe - literally: "I am no good to myself or anyone else. This is not fun." We'd gone through four mattresses trying to find one that was comfortable for me. I couldn't sleep because of the pain from the fibromyalgia, yet I was always exhausted and trying to sleep. It was a horrible and vicious circle. I screamed out and said: "Listen, I'm out of here. I feel like I'm going to die anyway, so it's not going to take much to just not wake up one day. Either You tell me how to get well so I can get back into my life and continue on my mission to help people, or I'm leaving. This is wasting time." Within two days, I was driving with one of my husband's clients up to the mountains to see another chiropractor. She wanted to stop at a health food store I had never even noticed before. I walked in and all of the flyers describing my problems were right there in front of me on a kiosk. Within two months, I was completely cured.

It happened quickly, but my protocol wasn't easy. It was a matter of changing my diet, changing my routine, clearing the toxins from my physical system, and learning what was going on inside my psyche. I realized that I had to find the "wholistic" cause(s) that was/were causing the pain, fatigue, loss of memory, fuzzy thinking, and finally my hair loss.

Louise Hay has a wonderful little book that's been out for many years.[1] I happened to look up Chronic Fatigue Syndrome and it said that CFS is an inner battle between dependence and independence. My mommy taught me I was going to go to college, be a sorority girl, meet my husband, and live happily ever after with kids,... and be taken care of. I hated the sorority. I didn't fit in. I lived in the library because I continued with a master's and PhD. I never really dated anybody steadily in college. The whole story was wrong. And then I ended up supporting my husband years later. I wanted to be taken care of, but I also wanted to be independent. You'll often see in chronic fatigue that there's that inner sense of: "I want to be able to relax and feel secure, but I want to do it my way on my own terms." Many of my clients with CFS and other conditions with fatigue relate to this issue.

The Illness

In my own case I chose a life without pain and suffering, so I took natural steps to get well. My troubles had begun, it turns out, when one tooth cracked and I had it filled, and then another one on the opposite side did the same thing. Both of the cracks were deep enough that I ended up needing root canals and crowns in both of them. My memory is so foggy from that period that I don't quite remember which tooth caused the most suffering, but I realize that my autoimmune troubles began at the same time that I received the root canals. [Currently I use a holistic dentist who uses special techniques, does not use metal amalgams, and doesn't believe in root canals and crowns on dead teeth because they can be very detrimental to one's health.[2]]

---

[1] Hay, Louise.(1984) *Heal Your Body*. Carlsbad, CA: Hay House.

[2] For more information check out: Meinig, G.E., DDS, FACD (2008) *Root Canal Cover-Up: A Founder of the Association of Root Canal Specialists Discovers Evidence That Root Canals Damage Your Health – Learn What to Do.* La Mesa, CA: Price-Pottenger Nutrition Foundation.

At that time I was working hard to pay off loans we had taken for a move across the country, and to get my husband established in his chiropractic practice. There was a lot of stress in my own work schedule, and I was not getting enough exercise nor was I eating the healthy diet that I am now.

I gave up eating corn sometime around that period of my life, and that made a big difference, but I still enjoyed gluten and dairy – usually in the form of ice-cream. After a long work week my husband and I would reward ourselves with a big chocolate cake and lots of ice-cream on top. As much as I enjoyed that, it was starting to kill me.

The combination of my dental issues, high levels of stress, and bad diet (even though our diet was much better than the typical American usually eats) led to my development of an overgrowth of systemic candida. I became poisoned by the toxins generated by this gut flora overgrowth and that became the culprit that finally "broke the camel's back" so that I developed CFS and Fibromyalgia.

When I found the brochures exactly describing all of my symptoms, it was as though a miracle had happened and Heaven had sent me all of the answers that I needed. Now instead of treating the symptoms I could treat the causes. I chose the natural approach.

First I worked with a chiropractor who used applied and clinical kinesiology. With these techniques he knew what my body needed for my glandular as well as structural re-balancing. He also provided me with homeopathic remedies to kill the candida overgrowth and herbs to clear the residue from my body as it was destroyed.[3]

In the meantime I chose a diet that stopped feeding the candida and provided me with exactly what my body craved. Basically I went on a modified Paleo diet that consisted of eating meat and vegetables, with organic virgin olive oil if I wanted to create a stir-fry. I gave up all grains, dairy, fruits, sauces, and only used salt,

---

[3] For more information check out: Crook, William G., MD. (1986) *The Yeast Connection – A Medical Breakthrough: If You Feel Sick All Over, This Book Could Change Your Life.* Jackson, TN: Professional Books.

pepper, herbs, and lemon juice to flavor my meat and vegetables. This was not a difficult diet when I was at home cooking for myself, but when I was at work and ate in restaurants or university cafeterias it became much more difficult. I was diligent because I realized two things: 1- if I cheated, the chemical balance I was creating would be jeopardized, and 2- if I cheated the excruciating pain and other symptoms would return. I stuck to my protocol.

During this time I worked on my own to come to grips with my inner "tug of war" around independence or dependence, and I realized that since I was a better business person than my husband, and I was the one who really wanted a higher level lifestyle with choices, that I should just let go of my mother's promises and make it happen for myself... and that is exactly what I did once I made that decision.

After exactly two months I was symptom-free, twenty pounds lighter, and my energy had returned. I had a new lease on life and I knew what my body needed to be balanced. I had chosen life and it was returned to me. From that time through the present I have been sharing my story and coaching others to have hope that they can recuperate from autoimmune like I did.

My Practice

For the last 31 years, I've been studying and integrating energy therapy and energy medicine into my practice. Several years ago when I started attracting many people with autoimmune disorders, I decided these people are so sick that I absolutely need to know more than energy therapy, energy medicine, and energy psychology in order to work with the healing of their physical bodies. So I started another doctorate in Classical Naturopathy. I am now a Certified Natural Health Professional, almost a Doctor of Naturopathy, and almost a Certified Nutritional Counselor. I enjoy using whatever I learn with my clients, and I continue to see positive results in their cases.

In autoimmune cases, we are talking about serious conditions where one can't just say: "Oh well, the doctor said get off of gluten. I'll just take this little pill so I won't get affected by the gluten and I'm going to keep on eating it." Forget that concept. Gluten can actually lead to autoimmune disorders in many cases.

You don't have to test for Celiac disease to be very gluten intolerant or sensitive.[4] Diet is a major aspect of every autoimmune disorder, and in order for me to understand that better to help my clients, I needed to study more about in-depth nutrition and natural physical healing.

Our Western medicine masks symptoms so that people will not feel them and so that the pharmaceutical industry can sell drugs to make more money. The system is wonderful in giving our society what it wants, which is not to change one's style of life or diet. People have the attitude that they want to go on living exactly the way they've lived -that made them sick - so drugs mask the pain... but the source of the symptom may remain and will shift to another level of destruction in the body until it again gains attention. The body simply continues to try and balance itself in order to survive, so when drugs are introduced, not only is the original antigen or toxin still present, but now there are additional chemical agents requiring more balancing energy. This is why I choose the natural route to health in my own body and I endorse it with my clients.

What I see in many of my clients that are so very sick is that the emotional or causal energy that we shift vibrates at a higher frequency than our denser and slower vibrational physical bodies. The physical is generally the last part to heal in the process. I decided in my work with autoimmune clients that I need more tools to help the physical body "catch up" in the healing process with the emotional or "electrical/ energetic" body. I need a scope of practice that will allow me to go in and help the body speed up the rebalancing process so it can get well more quickly.

Each body is absolutely unique, so a practitioner needs to treat it uniquely. One can't just take something "off the shelf" and use it, because every case is different. I work with each unique person based on that person's history, family of origin, ancestry, past lives if they're into that, and also what's appearing within each session... using a "wholistic" approach.

---

[4] For more information check out: Korn, Danna. (2010) *Living Gluten-Free for Dummies*. 2nd Edition. Hoboken, NJ: John Wiley & Sons Publishers.

What Is Autoimmunity?

I have found in my many years of dealing with autoimmune disorders, that one of the key things going on when the body is beating up on itself, which is a basic description of autoimmune, is the inner war. Of top priority is our need to identify and clear our issues as we support our bodies by creating peace inside. In this book we're going to get into the case details of what this strange animal called autoimmune is. Some people think autoimmune is what we have in our body as our immune system. No – the immune system supports the safety and ultimate healing of the body, while in autoimmune disorders the immune system goes out of whack, attacking the body itself. The symptoms described in this book will show you the many faces of autoimmune and how each is unique and also similar.

Focusing on peace, inner compassion, clearing the inner critical voice, being conscious of how we treat ourselves, listening to the body when it speaks, is all serious stuff when it comes to autoimmune, and each case will show how we strive first to start creating peace so that the body can begin to re-balance, which is what it does so much better than being sick.[5]

The numbers that I have heard are that between 50 and 85 million Americans currently suffer from diagnosed autoimmune disorders. Right now, more and more degenerative, chronic diseases and conditions are being classified as autoimmune. Things that maybe in the past we didn't think were autoimmune are being put into that category now. That doesn't even include the many, many chronic conditions that are undiagnosed at this point, or the conditions that MDs feel are un-diagnosable. You'll notice many new names for symptoms that just basically describe the condition or pathology. This describing of the symptoms does not focus on the cause of the symptoms as we focus in both Energy Psychology and Naturopathy.

In autoimmune conditions a form of suicide is happening, except it's not a logical decision. The body, rather than the mind, is saying:

---

[5] Also check out: Graham, Linda. (2013) *Bouncing Back: Rewiring Your Brain for Maximum Resilience and Well-Being*. Novato, CA: New World Library.

"I've had enough. You're not listening. I'm speaking a language and you don't know it yet, and you had better notice or I'm out of here." Unfortunately, when we're born we're not issued a **Human Body 101** manual.[6] We really don't know how to listen to the body. The body is always giving us information and sharing clues to its health,... and, it doesn't know how to be sick,... period. The body is a wonderful organism that is constantly rebalancing itself in many, many ways – so many that we'll never even be able to fathom them. When we overload the body with toxic emotions or toxic air or water or food or GMOs or something else, the body only knows how to rebalance itself. Its bottom line is to survive and thrive.

"Of the 50 million* Americans living and coping with autoimmune disease (AD), more than 75 percent of them are women."[7]

"5-10% of any population, most of them women, can expect to suffer f rom an autoimmune disease in a lifetime."[8]

AUTOIMMUNE can be defined as the following:

- Noun: a condition in which the body produces an immune response against its own tissue constituents
- Adj: of, relating to, or caused by antibodies or T cells that attack molecules, cells, or tissues of the organism producing them[9]

- "White blood cells in the body's immune system help protect against harmful substances such as: bacteria, viruses, toxins, cancer cells, blood and tissue from outside the body. These substances contain antigens against which the immune system

---

[6] This is definitely a catchy title, but in my opinion, no human will ever know enough to do it justice... the body is miraculously complex.
[7] American Autoimmune Related Diseases Association. (2015) "Autoimmune Disease in Women; Autoimmunity: A Major Women's Health Issue". Eastpointe, MI: http://aarda.org https://www.aarda.org/autoimmune-information/autoimmune-disease-in-women   *(Some sources report up to 85 million Americans have now been diagnosed with autoimmune issues.)
[8] Anderson, Warwick, and Ian R. Mackay. (2014) *Intolerant Bodies: A Short History of Autoimmunity*. Baltimore, MD: John Hopkins University Press. (page 2)
[9] Pease, Roger W., Jr., Editor. (2006*) Merriam-Webster's Medical Dictionary*. Springfield, MA: Merriam-Webster, Inc.

produces antibodies that enable it to destroy these harmful substances.

- When you have an autoimmune disorder, your immune system does not distinguish between healthy tissue and antigens; as a result, the body sets off a reaction that destroys normal tissues."[10]

Some of the common Autoimmune Diseases include the following:

- Type 1 diabetes is now considered autoimmune;
- Rheumatoid arthritis;
- All the types of arthritis;
- Mono and Chronic fatigue, of course;
- Fibromyalgia;
- Crohn's disease is very serious;
- All the thyroid conditions: hyper-, hypo-, Graves', Hashimoto's;
- MS / Multiple Sclerosis;
- Lupus Erythematosus;
- Many skin conditions: eczema, psoriasis, hives, boils, acne.

And, not-so-common conditions, over 100 total, are also placed into the autoimmune category. Some of these are: Addison's Disease, Lou Gehrig's disease = Amyotrophic Lateral Sclerosis (ALS), Myasthenia gravis, Pernicious anemia, Sjogren's syndrome, among many others.

---

[10] See more at: MedlinePlus. (*2015*) "Autoimmune Diseases", *MedlinePlus: Trusted Health Information for You*.
http://www.nlm.nih.gov/medlineplus/autoimmunediseases.html

The Medical Doctor's Dilemma

Doctors traditionally have had so much trouble treating these disorders because they don't know the cause, so they can't treat it and allow the body to heal. If you delve in deeper and know a little bit more about the WHOLE person, such as in Energy Psychology or Naturopathy, often the emotional or energetic cause of why the body is attacking itself becomes apparent and obvious. In identifying and clearing or changing that, the body can start to rebalance.

In his book, *When the Body Says No: The Cost of Hidden Stress – Exploring the Stress-Disease Connection*, practicing physician, Dr. Gabor Mate' points out via his own case studies how many people with serious diseases and disorders appear to similarly hold emotional scars from their earlier lives. He woefully recounts many patients who died because traditional medicine could not treat the perceived emotional cause of their sickness. As a maverick in his own traditional medical profession his books and newsletter span a wide range of conditions and cases.

In chapter one of *When the Body Says No*, he enthusiastically quotes a letter written by Dr. Noel B. Hershfield, clinical professor of medicine at the University of Calgary:

> "The new discipline of psychoneuroimmunology has now matured to the point where there is compelling evidence, advanced by scientists from many fields, that an intimate relationship exists between the brain and the immune system... An individual's emotional makeup, and the response to continued stress may indeed be causative in the many diseases that medicine treats but whose [origin] is not yet known–diseases such as scleroderma, and the vast majority of rheumatic disorders, the inflammatory bowel disorders, diabetes, multiple sclerosis, and legions of other conditions which are represented in each medical subspecialty."[11]

---

[11] Mate', Gabor, MD. (2011) *When the Body Says No: The Cost of Hidden Stress – Exploring the Stress-Disease Connection*. Hoboken, NJ: John Wiley & Sons. Chapter One.

Dr. Mate' continues in his own words to state:

> "The surprising revelation in this letter was the existence of a new field of medicine. What is psychoneuroimmunology? As I learned, it is no less than the science of the interactions of mind and body, the indissoluble unity of emotions and physiology in human development and throughout life in health and illness. That dauntingly complicated word means simply that this discipline studies the ways that the psyche – the mind and its content of emotions — profoundly interacts with the body's nervous system and how both of them, in turn, form an essential link with our immune defenses. Some have called this new field psychoneuroimmunoendocrinology to indicate that the endocrine, or hormonal, apparatus is also a part of our system of whole body response. Innovative research is uncovering just how these links function all the way down to the cellular level. We are discovering the scientific basis of what we have known before and have forgotten, to our great loss."[12]

In just these two paragraphs, Dr. Mate' not only introduces the relatively new field of scientific study, psychoneuroimmunology, which focuses on the connection of the mind with the body's physiology, but endorses the argument that emotional issues or traumas can cause dis-ease including autoimmune disorders. Although traditional medicine has yet to incorporate the findings into practice, the field of Energy Psychology focuses on clearing the emotional issues or blockages using a variety of approaches, and clinical studies have shown that in doing so, the body's physiology then can over time return to natural homeostasis. I highly endorse Dr. Mate's writings and presentations as he continues to enlighten the medical community as well as the general public.[13]

---

[12] Mate', Gabor, MD. (2011) *When the Body Says No: The Cost of Hidden Stress – Exploring the Stress-Disease Connection*. Hoboken, NJ: John Wiley & Sons. Chapter One.
[13] Check out his TEDX Talk here: http://drgabormate.com

Blocks in the Path of Healing

A typical, across-the-board symptom of most autoimmune conditions is depression. Much is being taken away from people suffering from autoimmune, or much has already been lost. They're very sad and frustrated. They don't like their new lives. Some of them don't want to go forward because they don't want to have lost everything that they've lost. Many of them are very foggy in their minds. Whether they've been diagnosed with chronic fatigue or something else, they're often very exhausted all the time, and don't know why they have no pep, no zest, no passion for life.

We've heard it from all different sources that if the environment doesn't change, then whatever you do with a client or patient is not going to work. You can't change something and let it go right back into the hurtful environment and then expect any changed results. And, the same goes with autoimmune or any other disease or chronic condition. Life changes must be made in order for healing to take place and to maintain. And, this is very difficult for people living in a culture where every illness begs for it's magic pill for instant cure.

In any practice of any discipline there can be blocks to healing, and as an "energy detective" I like to search these out as I work with clients. Here are some examples of difficult cases where some things that needed to change just would not budge, so the end results were less than the potential.

The Power of Expectations:

Case I:
In one of my autoimmune cases a 21-year-old client was suffering from acute Crohn's Disease. He was diagnosed at a young age and had been suffering ever since. When he entered my practice he weighed 84 pounds, and still lived at home with his parents because he was too sick to take care of himself. In Crohn's Disease, which is an inflammation of the gastro-intestinal tract, the symptoms are the following:
- Persistent Diarrhea.
- Rectal bleeding.
- Urgent need to move bowels.

- Abdominal cramps and pain.
- Sensation of incomplete evacuation.
- Constipation

Before getting pregnant with this boy his mother had had a miscarriage, and during the second pregnancy she held extreme fear that death or something horrible would be wrong with the baby, or that the baby would have physical problems. Combine this with an overbearing father who pushes to get things done and has little patience for chronic conditions such as his son exhibits.

In the womb the developing child picks up the fears and emotions of the mother. Potentially, it was this mom's emotional mind-set and expectations while in the womb that her highly sensitive son lived up to, reflecting multiple physical problems his whole life, finally leading to Crohn's Disease. And, while both parents love him dearly, his father's regular comments: "If I were you, I'd be well by now. Why aren't you doing this? You should be doing that," cause anger and exacerbate the Crohn's symptoms.

Both parents are usually at home with their son, and the three-way dynamics with both parents projecting their expectations on this sensitive and very ill young man may block the way to healing. He feels like a perpetual failure as he continues to try and please both parents, but angry outbursts often lead to back-slides in any health gains he has made. Until the home dynamics change dramatically, this boy cannot heal even though he is applying multiple approaches that generally work with other clients. He can't escape the dynamic because he is afraid to leave the house. He's afraid he'll have a diarrhea attack. This is no way to live, and it points out why so many autoimmune sufferers become hopeless. They can't stand living in their bodies. The symptoms are so horrible, and often the causes are even worse.

Case II:
In another case I had a very educated man who held a doctorate in biological sciences who claimed: "I'm going to prove to the medical community that I'm going to get over Hashimoto's (a thyroid disorder). My mother had that diagnosis. I had that diagnosis. I'm going to show them I can do it naturally." I'm thinking: "No pressure, right?" I've already mentioned a correlation between Type

A personalities and autoimmune disorders, and this seemed to be a classic case.

We have to remember that the body is in charge – not the logical mind. No matter what the client wants to have as a priority, it'll be successful only if it is the body's priority. There are no "one-minute miracles" in clearing autoimmune, unless the body has done all its rebalancing and the only thing left is the final emotional piece of the puzzle that you're working with on that particular day. I have witnessed some miracles with my clients, but it usually takes about four or five sessions. Since an autoimmune condition took a long time to develop, it's not going to be cured overnight. Right?

Psychological Reversal

In Energy Psychology there is a known state of mind that can block the path of healing. This "psychological reversal" occurs when a person is so dogmatically positioned against something that they literally block it from working.

One case of this that sometimes shows up in my practice is when a person simply does not believe in energy or Energy Psychology or the body's electro-magnetic biofield or its meridian system. By actively not believing that something will work can absolutely block its effectiveness.

Another example is when a medical doctor has given a dire prognosis of a "life sentence of suffering" and the client believes everything told to him or her by an MD, so that person simply expects to stay sick and suffer.

Yet another example of psychological reversal is when the root cause of a disorder is so traumatic that PTSD/ Post Traumatic Stress Disorder has set in, and that person's subconscious mind believes on some level that in remembering or talking about the trauma they will actually die. Even though this doesn't make logical sense, the subconscious mind is much more powerful than the conscious mind, and it remains in charge of such things.

There are a number of energy therapy techniques that can be used to clear all forms of psychological reversal, so if a person is willing to work with me, we can usually get beyond these blocks.

History & Possible Causes of Autoimmune

John Hopkins University puts out a series of books, each focused on different diseases and categories of diseases and their histories. In a new 2014 text by Warwick Anderson & Ian Mackay called *Intolerant Bodies – A Short History of Autoimmunity*[14], the researchers cite the history of autoimmune symptoms or conditions through the ages and through many philosophies of health and healing treatments over time, many of which did not recognize the conditions as actually the body hurting itself. The book is quite interesting and shows how little we knew before and how quickly this field of study is gaining momentum.

I like Charles Rosenberg's Foreword in the book where he states:
> "The phenomenon of autoimmunity recalls an older way of thinking about the fundamental nature of disease, a way of thinking that was commonplace in 1800 but marginal by 2000. Two centuries ago the occurrence of disease is ordinarily understood by both physicians and laymen as an individual, physiological response to an individual's unique bodily makeup and life course. Diet and exercise interacting with physical environment, life circumstances and constitutional endowment resulted in sickness or health."[15]

He goes on to say:
> "As the body moved through time it was continuously self-regulating, adjusting and readjusting and thus always at risk. In this traditional and nonspecific way of thinking about disease there was little role for infection and infectious agents.
>
> One might describe this way of thinking about the nature and origin of disease as holistic and physiological, as well as cumulative and biographical. The phenomenon of

---

[14] Anderson, Warwick, and Ian R. Mackay. (2014) *Intolerant Bodies: A Short History of Autoimmunity*. Baltimore, MD: John Hopkins University Press.

[15] Charles E. Rosenberg – "Foreword" for: Anderson, Warwick, and Ian R. Mackay. (2014) *Intolerant Bodies: A Short History of Autoimmunity*. Baltimore, MD: John Hopkins University Press. (page xii)

autoimmunity, with its implied juxtaposition of biological individuality and particular circumstance, reminds us of this older, integrative way of seeing the body in time and in terms of its cumulative interaction with itself and with its external – yet internalized – environment."[16]

Looking at the whole picture is what Naturopathy still does, but often the medical profession overlooks. Naturopaths don't look at putting people in a box with a percentage of other people that report with similar symptoms. They say, "This is a unique body, unique experience, a unique soul, maybe with unique past lives, obviously unique heredity, etc. So let's treat this person very specifically for who he or she really is instead of making him or her a number with many others."

Another good point in the last paragraph of the quote: "…this way of thinking about the nature and origin of disease as holistic and physiological, as well as cumulative and biographical," shows the difference between the philosophy and approach to disease at that time, compared with where medicine went after that stage, starting in the 1900's or even in the late 1800's, where germ theory become the prevailing philosophy. Rather than considering that a symptom relates to the natural rebalancing of the body, in germ theory an outside "alien" comes into the body and the healing approach is to fight it off.   Why haven't they found a cure for the common cold? The common cold is not just a bug flying by. It's the body rebalancing. Yes, you're going to have symptoms because you've done something, you've gotten into something, and the body needs to purge. The natural health, energy medicine, and naturopathic physicians still think of the whole person, and that's what I urge you to do when you're considering autoimmune and its treatment.

The authors go on to say:

> "Until late in the nineteenth century, most medical doctors – and most of their patients – regarded disease as a

---

[16] Charles E. Rosenberg – "Foreword" for: Anderson, Warwick, and Ian R. Mackay. (2014) *Intolerant Bodies: A Short History of Autoimmunity*. Baltimore, MD: John Hopkins University Press. (page xii)

disturbance of an individual's constitutional equilibrium."[17] It's all about balance, whether it's balancing the emotions, the self-compassion, the body, the intake, the out-take, it's very important. The body is in a constant state of flux where there is a balancing act of: circumstances, habits, background, nature, nurture, what we're born with in our DNA, what our predispositions to disease are, and the stressors that trigger things. We all carry the predisposition to multiple types of disease in our human genes. We know now that stress levels trigger these to activate and create the dis-ease in our lives. If we don't trigger the predisposition, it stays dormant. Bruce Lipton and Candace Pert both discuss this from different scientific approaches.[18]

We may say here that an opposite state to stress is happiness. When the dopamine, serotonin, and oxytocin endorphins or "happy hormones" are flowing through our systems we don't feel stressed and the dormant dis-ease predispositions remain dormant.

Mark Leary is a Professor of Psychology at Duke University. His audio series with study guide text, *Understanding the Mysteries of Human Behavior*, states: "Research suggests that only about 10 percent of people's happiness is due to their life circumstance and that about 50 percent of it is due to people's genetic makeup."[19] Then he goes on to say, because he's a traditional psychologist, that 10 percent is life situation, and 40 percent is due to intentional behavior. This refers to the people we choose to be around, the lifestyle we choose, and other conscious choices. That's all fine and dandy in a Pollyanna kind of world, but let's look at all the other real-life occurrences in a wholistic way. What happens when a

---

[17] Anderson, Warwick, and Ian R. Mackay. (2014) *Intolerant Bodies: A Short History of Autoimmunity*. Baltimore, MD: John Hopkins University Press. (page 3)

[18] I highly recommend books by both scientists including the following: Lipton, Bruce H., Ph.D. (2008) 2nd Edition. *The Biology of Belief: Unleashing the Power of Consciousness, Matter & Miracles*. Hay House Publishers: www.hayhouse.com -and- Pert, Candace B., Ph.D. (1997) *Molecules of Emotion: The Science Behind Mind-Body Medicine*. New York, NY: Scribner.

[19] Leary, Mark, Ph.D. (2012). *Understanding the Mysteries of Human Behavior*: Course Guidebook & Audio. Chantilly, VA: The Great Courses Publishers.

person is in the womb of their mother who experiences something emotional, and the baby's subconscious and whole viscera including all energy meridians takes on everything she feels? What happens when that baby is born and experiences the trauma of that birth action? And then, how about the emotions that the small child picks up just like a sponge up to the age of 7 through 12 when his cognitive brain comes online and he finally realizes he is separate and not just part of his mother and everything around him? When that child is in school, everything he notices and feels is taken in by his subconscious which just goes: "Yes, yes, yes," claiming them to belong to him and his own experience. There is no conscious choice in this real scenario that happens with all of us, so this distorts Leary's percentages.

What we see in some cases is that memories may come up in psychological sessions such as abuse, abandonment, loss, betrayal, and other traumas, but they may be second-hand events that actually happened to someone else, but a person's subconscious via the process just described, took it on as his own memory and held onto the emotional stress. Even these "non-local", "second-hand" emotions need to be cleared in order to avert the stress that may eventually lead to dis-ease of some kind. Taking this into consideration, Mark Leary's numbers stating that 10 percent of people's happiness is due to life experience and 40 percent is due to intentional behavior seems way off because so much of our experience is unintentionally taken on from others' experiences.

This just goes to show that looking at possible causes and probabilities based on stressors coming from similar but different treatment vantage points can lead to many different hypotheses of the root cause of a disorder and then how to treat it. You will learn by experiencing each of the subsequent case studies in this book how I wholistically approach each client and treat them with natural tools.

Tips for Healthy Living

Before getting into the cases I want to share the natural protocol tips that every person in a body needs to remember as we're keeping ourselves healthy, getting healthier, or supporting the body to rebalance and detox.

As part of my doctorate studies in Naturopathy I earned my Certification as a Natural Health Professional. During an intensive eight-day training program for this CNHP credential we covered many kinds of wholistic and natural approaches to helping the body stay in balance or rebalance.

I have chosen here to share with you a list of things that are very paramount in keeping a healthy body. Whether you're already suffering from something or you are still in a healthy body, in order to keep it healthy I'm sharing 17 different points that you need to know. These are not necessarily things that you'll get from your medical doctor or from another practitioner. Pulled from a compilation of different disciplines, you can bring the information from this section into your life to help support your health or to help support you to get healthy.

In illness of all kinds your body shows certain symptoms and we're working to clear the causes of those symptoms so the body can rebalance. The 17 points I'm sharing here are things you can start integrating. You don't need a practitioner to do most of them; you can do them on your own. Some of them may take a little stretch from you, and some of them may not. You can allow your body to stay in balance naturally if you keep the following points in mind.

Human Body 101

Did you know that your body doesn't really know how to be sick? The body is a miraculous, wonderful organism. I won't compare it to a mechanical computer, although a computer has a lot of energy in it that goes beyond just the bits and pieces and the mechanics of it. The body is way beyond a computer, and it works faster and better. It only gets "sick" because it is out of balance. When you suffer from the "common cold" and when you get diarrhea or nausea, or start having mucus coming out of your nose, it is usually a way that the body is detoxing. When you focus on stopping all the symptoms, then the body can't drain the toxins, so you're stuck with the toxins inside longer than they need to be there.

Your body replaces all of its cells every 90 to 100 days, so 180 days from now, if you are careful about what you do for your body, you will be living in a totally different body with different cells. Just imagine it. This includes brain cells and all of the other cells in your body; they regenerate. So, in order to nurture these cells, we need to maintain them and the whole body via these 17 points I'm sharing.

Like the full body, each cell requires that it be fed with the right balance of nutrients, hydrated, allowed to eliminate waste, and cleansed of the waste in the environment. In order to support our cells to do this you need to be aware of how to keep the cells and full body in balance. The following points will help you as you maintain living in our modern and toxed-out society

The Seventeen Points

Some of these points are going to be review for you. Some of them may be new material to consider. Each refers to an important part of your life, and when you keep the tenet in mind you will feel the results of a body maintaining balance.

Point #1 – Healthy Air

Air quality is so very important to your health and well-being, and how you breathe is also something to be aware of.

Back in grad school I had an apartment that was close to a neighboring gas station. When my windows were open I could smell the gas fumes and I realized they made me dizzy, and I felt like I needed to sleep a lot. Heavy metal poisoning can come from breathing toxic air like gas fumes. If you live close to an airport, you may have airplanes dumping fuel as they circle the airport, or if it's an Air Force base or other military base, often they have too much fuel and don't want to land with that much so they fuel up in the air. If you're walking down the street and there's a plane overhead getting ready to land, you may smell the petroleum.

You've got to be aware of what you're breathing. Toxic fumes in the environment can definitely impact your health or lack thereof. I'm a little concerned about my own beautiful cabin sitting up on a mountain that I heat with two propane gas log fireplaces plus a central HVAC system. I don't really know for sure how healthy the propane fumes are for me and my particular lungs. Look around your environment. Make sure that whenever it's a nice day out that you breathe fresh air.

Air is really important. Often when I facilitate energy therapy sessions I get into deep breathing. I ask clients to breathe in a deep sense of peace or health and to hold it in, and then breathe it out and feel it leaving their lungs along with the blocked energy. Just by focusing on the breath during meridian tapping or while using other energy therapy techniques can make a profound difference.

But, often people just breathe in the top of their lungs. Shallow breathing does not provide the oxygen that our cells need. All of our cells need that oxygen. Without it, they're going to die and then we're going to get sick. Good air and good breathing techniques make a huge difference, and that is why yoga is such a potent practice. It teaches how to breathe deeply. Pilates, when done correctly, is also a really wonderful exercise practice. Neither one of these are too energetic, yet both provide the body with the necessary oxygen that it needs. If you're in a weakened condition, you can do things like yoga or pilates. Qigong and other kinds of martial arts kinds of exercises are also wonderful in that they teach you to breathe. Your body needs good, fresh air, and it needs lots of it. Start to practice breathing in a full breath so that your stomach even goes out and you feel your lungs totally filling up. See how long you can hold each breath in your lungs and then breathe it completely out. See if you can hold your lungs totally empty for a little while before you breathe back in.

Point #2 – Good Food

You have probably heard too much about diets. I have a number of points that I will list about my recommendations for "good" food diets. The best rule is to remember that everything that enters your body is either beneficial or harmful – except for good water, which is neutral.

- A first suggestion that I have for everyone is to get off of "Round-up" crops. Any crop that has become immune to this potent herbicide is automatically presenting a genetic modification into your system that can wreak havoc with your gastro-intestinal flora as well as your immune system. Another way of looking at this is to eat only Organic or Non-GMO (genetically-modified) foods.

- Good oils are very important to any diet regime, and if you cut out oils or fat you will find it very difficult to eliminate and to assimilate your nutrients. Any partially or hydrogenated oils such as are used in pre-packed pastries, grocery store bakery items, or other off-the-shelf foods are non-digestible and are made for a long shelf life, which does not aid in your digestion process.

- With my autoimmune clients I endorse a modified Paleo-type diet without gluten and dairy, and with very few grains. There are many reasons why gluten is dangerous for the body, and often getting it out of your diet can seem difficult. There are many resources available to help in this.[20]

- It's also important to keep in mind a balance between the alkaline-ash-producing foods and the acid-ash-creating foods that you intake.[21] This is all related to pH, which we're going to get into in a little bit. Foods need to supply good health and they need to provide a good balance of your pH in your body. Whenever you go to a swimming pool, you would hope that the lifeguard there or the owner of the pool keeps the pH correct. If not, your skin may burn or break out because the water is too alkaline or too acid. Either way, you may get sick because if the pH is not right, it can grow microbes that can be destructive when out-of-balance in your system. When this happens the water starts getting foggy, or full of algae, and you won't want to swim there. pH balance is also why you have to test aquarium water. Fish

---

20 See: Korn, Danna. (2010) *Living Gluten-Free for Dummies*. 2nd Edition. Hoboken, NJ: John Wiley & Sons Publishers.
21 Learn more from: Toney, T. (2010). *Get Clean Go Green EcoDiet: The Secrets of an Alkaline Environment.* USA: New Earth Publishers.

die if the pH isn't correct. Our bodies also die if the pH isn't correct. In fact, we cannot assimilate vitamins and minerals and nutrients if our body is not in the right pH range. You may be taking many vitamins every single day, but your body may not be assimilating any of them if your pH is not correct.

- Many people endorse 80 percent raw and 20 percent cooked foods, and at least 80 percent natural, fresh foods, even if you cook them. None of us really should be eating refined foods. Anything that has a whole list of ingredients, including chemicals, colors, flavorings are considered "fake" foods, and your body doesn't need them. Any kind of refined flours are also not good for your body because the nutrients have probably been refined out of them.

- Many people are becoming allergic to all grains, but do not fear, nut flours and natural seeds are amply available for cooking, baking, and using in all the ways that grain flours have been applied in the past. You don't have to eat the typical foods that you've always eaten in order to get your favorite dishes with your favorite flavors. Good food is really important.

Point #3 – Good Water

When I discuss "good water", I'm talking about a limited kind of water. We're talking water that is the best for you and your cells. That water is either distilled water or reverse osmosis water. Many people argue that the distilled has no minerals in it and all the good things have been completely vaporized out. The interesting thing I learned was when you have natural spring water or even typical well water full of natural minerals, the body cannot deal with these inorganic minerals, the ones that are minute particles of rocks, sand, and that come out of the earth. They're wonderful but the body cannot assimilate them directly. If they go through a plant and a plant takes the minerals up through the soil and into its roots and then we eat the plant or the fruit from the plant, then we can get the minerals. They then become organic minerals instead of inorganic minerals, and our body can assimilate those. So, don't believe the argument that you have to have spring water with minerals – natural or added back in. Since we're not assimilating those anyway because they're inorganic, your body has to take extra energy to digest those and expel them. Again, reverse osmosis water or distilled water are the best waters to be drinking.

You are probably feeling dehydrated most of the time and don't even know it. Symptoms may include fatigue, fogginess, nausea, dizziness, listlessness, aches and pains, abdominal cramps, and I could go on. So, here is what you need to do in order to adequately hydrate your cells so they can function in a healthy manner. Take your body weight and divide that in half. This number in ounces is the amount of good water your body should be drinking each day. For example, if you weigh 100 pounds, divide that by two, which is 50. You should be drinking 50 ounces of good water per day. And, good water does not mean coffee, tea, juice, or anything except water. And, then, after doing energy therapy work, when I remind you to: "Drink lots of water, more than you usually drink.," that means you're going to drink more water than your baseline because energy work takes more water. If you're not drinking enough daily good water, I highly recommend you change your ways. Your body needs this.

Point #4 - The Digestive Process

Yes, it does start in your mouth. That's why it's so important to chew your food. People suggest that your food should be a liquid before you even swallow it. If you're eating a few bites, chewing a few times and then swallowing a big lump like a dog, then it is more difficult and takes more energy for your body to digest it. We need to baby our digestive system because it is of paramount importance to our overall health and well-being. We need to take food into the mouth, let it go down into the stomach where it'll sit in the stomach for up to an hour or maybe more. Then it starts going into the small intestine. A lot has to occur in that digestive process. You really need to support your digestion. The best way to do that is to eat good foods.

You know that you don't want to eat huge quantities of protein from meat. You also don't want to cut good fats out of your diet. Anybody that's on a low-fat diet is hurting themselves. If it's good fat, you can eat all the coconut oil that you feel like eating and it's going to be good for you. You're not going to eat that much because it fills you up. It's nutritious and it tastes good. There's a certain point where you're just not going to want anymore. Don't cut fats out of your diet or else you won't be able to digest. Your body needs good, essential fatty acids.

Point #5 – "BULLS" of Elimination

Elimination is a big aspect of your digestive process, and this doesn't just include the intestines and eliminating through the bowels. That's just one part of a sophisticated and whole-body system. Elimination of toxins from the body is something that we have to keep in mind. Here is an overview of the different body processes that we must be aware of and that we need to maintain in order to eliminate the toxins that come out of every single cell in our body every day, multiple times every day. I want you to imagine the word bulls, "BULLS".

"B" is for bowels.
We eliminate via our intestines and colon or bowel. When we are healthy we eliminate two or three times a day depending on whether we eat two or three meals per day. We should have an elimination for every meal that we eat. That's normal. Hydration, the right vitamins and minerals in balance, and oils in our diet can aid this process. If you have trouble there may be nutritional, emotional, toxic, or structural reasons why you have difficulty eliminating, and a functional medical doctor or naturopathic physician can look at your full wholistic profile and help you to understand how to remedy your situation.

"U" stands for your urinary tract.
It is not just the water that goes through you. When you are taking your vitamins and you urinate and it's very yellow, that is a normal cycle of the Vitamin B coming through you because it only stays in your system for six hours and then leaves naturally. If it hasn't been absorbed in around six hours, it's eliminated and that's why you need to keep taking your multiple B vitamins. Normal urine should look like a light wheat yellow color if it's healthy. Different people urinate with different frequency. When you are eating a healthy diet urination shouldn't burn. If your urine burns, that may mean that your urine is too acid or too alkaline indicating an imbalance in your pH, or that you may have some level of irritation

or infection in the urinary tract. Basically the urinary system gets rid of the toxins or wastes released from your intestines and processed via the kidneys and bladder. It's a wonderful way to help eliminate many different things from the body that it doesn't need.

"L" is for lungs - another way that our body eliminates toxins.

Every time you breathe out carbon dioxide, you're also breathing out toxins from the cells. When your red blood cells that carry the nutrients and oxygen go through your lungs and you take a deep breath of air, you're breathing in oxygen. It goes into the red blood cells and then is carried by your cardiovascular system to deliver the oxygen to every cell in your body. As it delivers the oxygen then the blood cell picks up the CO_2, the carbon dioxide, which is the waste from the cell having already used the oxygen. The oxygenated blood leaves the lungs via the arteries and then the CO_2-filled cells return to the lungs via the veins to be expelled. When you breathe out, you expel many toxins that come out of the blood. What an amazing and intricate system of cleansing this is that includes both the vascular and respiratory systems!

When you exercise aerobically and start breathing deeply and taking full breaths of air – also when you do yoga or Pilates and you take deep breaths, your lungs are expelling more of the toxic refuse from your cells. That's good for you because while you are de-toxing you're also energizing yourself by getting more oxygen into your cells. That gives you much more energy.

The second "L" stands for the lymph system.

The lymph system, like the blood system, takes toxins away from the cells. The lymph system also takes the nutrition to the cells, just like the blood system. The lymph system is kind of like a sister system, and it is connected with the neuro-lymphatic rubbing points that we will refer to later. The lymph system is also where the lymphocytes or white blood cells are manufactured and through which they are delivered into the vascular system. Lymph is thought of as being more of a clear fluid that flows throughout the body. This system has no heart to pump it through the body; instead the flow is maintained by action from your big muscles. The only way your lymph system is very active is when you move. The more movement you do, the healthier your lymph system is. Your lymph can then take the beneficial substances to the cells to feed them with nutrition and take away the waste. There's elimination from every single cell in our human form, and the waste, which is toxic to our body, is taken away in the lymph. Then it is actually placed into the bowels through the intestines or into the kidneys and bladder, and you expel it through urine. The lymph system is so very important.

When you hear somebody with breast cancer and they've got lymph nodes that are involved and they have all those cut out, they've got a problem. Those lymph nodes are helpful to helping the whole lymph system in feeding the vital cells of the organs and all the tissues and all the cells in the body. You need your lymph system. In order to keep it healthy, you need to do some kind of movement or exercise each day. Your main lymph-related organ is your spleen. When people have accidents and then they have their spleen removed, the spleen makes the blood cells and supports the lymph system. We need our spleens just as we are meant to have all of our organs intact.

The final letter, "S", is for the skin.
When you sweat or perspire, you are also letting go of toxins. You may taste your sweat sometimes, and it might seem salty. That is letting go of the alkaline pH. Sometimes it may hold an odor or putrid taste, maybe like chemicals, because it's expelling toxins. Generally if your pH is balanced and you are healthy, you should not have bad body odor at all. You should not have to use any kind of deodorant if your diet is clean and your pH is balanced. I would never recommend using an antiperspirant because you want to perspire – it is the healthy thing that your body requires. Don't use something that keeps you from perspiring. Some people still need a deodorant, and there are natural, aloe-based options which will work well. If you have a strong body odor or you notice that your body odor changes, you need to look at what you're eating.

Point #6 - Essential Fatty Acids

There are a group of fatty acids that our body does not make and yet they are required in order for the body to be in balance and to function the way it needs to function. The fatty acids are considered to be Vitamin F. You get these essential fatty acids in fish oil. If you're taking a good fish oil or flax oil supplement daily, that's good.

Make sure that you're buying a good brand, not just a cheap, discount supplement. You get what you pay for. If you're getting the "big box store" brand or a generic brand, it's like going to a fast food take-out and buying a piece of meat versus going to a special restaurant where you can get grass-fed, organic, no hormone, wonderful, pampered beef and get a beautiful cut of steak. There's a difference in quality. You're going to get much more benefit from one versus the other. In fact, the other may not help you at all.

Point #7 – pH balance

I mentioned the importance of this already. pH stands for "potential hydrogen", and it relates to the body's ability to absorb minerals which are vital to survival. To stay alive your blood pH must fall between 7.35 and 7.45. Neutral is considered at 7. An optimal range for both urine and saliva should be between 6.3 and 6.6, with a rating of 6.4 considered best. If you stay within that range 6.3-6.6 you will be able to absorb and assimilate most supplements. Even if you're buying the right foods and vitamin supplements, your body can't use the nutrients therein if your pH is off. It's like your body is full of acid rain and that's not good.[22] In order to check your own level of health based on pH, you can go to your health food store and get some pH strips to test your urine and to test your saliva.

For example, in the case of many Thyroid conditions, both hyper- and hypo-, the digestive system may not have a healthy pH between 6.3 and 6.6, so it cannot assimilate iodine, which is important for this organ, and is a substance that can only be absorbed within this very narrow range. Some other vitamins and minerals have broader ranges, but that will not support the thyroid getting the iodine that it needs to function. This, along with other factors, can create an imbalance that will lead to dis-ease in the thyroid.

Without a proper pH balance, digestion and elimination are moving at the wrong speed which means even the best source of nutrients cannot be assimilated. Without nutrients, every system of the body will be incapable of functioning at 100%. When the pH is balanced,

---

[22] To learn more about this in easy-to-digest discussion, go to: Toney, T. (2010). *Get Clean Go Green EcoDiet: The Secrets of an Alkaline Environment*. USA: New Earth Publishers.

the rest of the body can achieve balance. Naturopaths can usually help you with pH balancing tests and information for your unique body.

Interestingly enough, there is a specific "fibromyalgia pattern" where the saliva pH is lower than (more acidic) than 6.4 and the urine pH is higher (more alkaline) than 6.4. Other indications are:
- blood anemia with deficiency in iron and/or in Vitamin B12,
- diarrhea if the acid number is very low,
- leg cramps indicating problems with calcium utilization,
- muscular discomfort in the lower extremities with aching bones, and
- this pattern can lead to strokes, high blood pressure, and vascular problems with vessel fragility.

Point #8 – Hygiene

Most everybody in our culture generally keeps pretty good hygiene, but do you realize how many poisons are in our clothes washing products, our soaps, our shampoos, our conditioners, our facial and body lotions, our lipsticks, our cosmetics, our air purifiers, our perfumes, our toilet paper? Look around you at all the products you're using for your personal hygiene and make sure that you're not poisoning yourself. When somebody comes to me and they say: I've got all these breakouts in a certain area of my body, I always ask them: "What are you using to wash your clothes? Are you using the strongest thing that's going to get out all the dirt? Are you using the cheapest brand on the market?" You don't want to do that. You want to make sure you're using good, healthy things that are not going to hurt your body. Everything that touches your skin immediately goes into your blood stream. You might say: "I've got thick skin." Right, but if you put a lotion on your skin, or if your skin is next to new clothes that haven't been washed and still have chemicals on them, you're taking in toxins right then and there. Your body has to expel those toxins immediately. It takes extra energy to do that. Just beware.

Point #9 – Exercise

This is so important to all of your systems, and as mentioned before, your lymph system depends on the movement of your big muscles like in exercise. You need to move your body. You need to keep your joints moving or else you will start to get still and lose range of motion. You need to keep your muscles moving or else they will quickly atrophy. Exercise doesn't need to be strenuous, but you need to move that lymph so that your cells can be fed and the toxins can be removed.

Point #10 – Good Sleep

If you have chronic fatigue, you may sleep a lot or be tired all the time and wish you could sleep all the time. If you suffer from fibromyalgia or chronic pain, maybe it's hard for you to sleep. A typical body needs at least seven to eight hours of sleep, not less. If you can't sleep a full seven or eight hours per night, you've got to look at what you're doing to keep yourself awake. Are you ingesting caffeine? Are you using nicotine? Are you using electronic devices late at night before you go to sleep? Are you watching scary movies or very upsetting things? Are you watching the news before you go to bed at night? Are you eating chocolate or drinking coffee in the afternoon or evening? Whatever it is, there's something keeping you awake. Is it just the stress, where you wake up in the middle of the night and all of a sudden you're so stressed out, you're making lists, having conversations with coworkers or your boss, or you're worried about your health condition, or about your finances?

There are many tools that can be used to help you claim quality sleep in the amounts that you need. The energy therapy meridian tapping can really help you to go to sleep. I would also advise that you do not look at computer screens, cell phone screens, TV screens, or anything bright and light for about an hour before you go to sleep if you're having problems sleeping. If caffeine may be your problem, stop eating that after noon. Take your caffeine in the morning if you have to have it at all.

Make sure that you get a good night's sleep. If you can, allow yourself to sleep until you wake up naturally. Don't set an alarm. If your body is tired, let it take a nap. Don't beat up on yourself because you need the nap. It doesn't mean you're lazy. If you suffer from autoimmune, you probably have a problem with your body, so let yourself sleep.

Point #11 - Emotional Balance

As an Energy Psychologist, I look first at a person's emotional balance when they present to me with a physical or other kind of problem. In autoimmune there is usually an emotional component stemming from earlier in life that needs to be addressed and the emotional charge cleared in order for the body to be able to move into full healing mode.

In my practice I use energy psychology tools including meridian tapping and pressure point holding, and naturopathy tools including homeopathics and flower essences to clear emotions having to do with the conditions presented, such as: fears, self doubts, pain, stress, and any other emotions involved. We must have emotions balanced in order for other treatments to work and to allow the body to rebalance. This step which is often overlooked, is so important.[23]

Point #12 - Spiritual Balance

Having a private spiritual life is vitally important to humans. Whatever you believe doesn't matter, whether you believe in the Universe or God or Jesus, you could be Buddhist or Muslim or Hindu or Christian or Jewish. It doesn't matter. You need to have a private, higher-than-third-dimensional connection. You could say it's with your Higher Self, your Guardian Angel, your God, your sense of the Creator, your sense of the Almighty Power. When you are connected, you can feel that sense of peacefulness. You can get a sense of inspiration and can let go of your worries. You can ask for help. That is vitally important to your whole self. If you're an atheist, look for something that you truly believe in. Focus on that. There is a god for you. Look at where you put your energy. What are your beliefs? What do you really stand for? Are you an earth lover? You may believe in the earth. You may believe in the earth spirits rather than God. That's fine. It doesn't matter, just have a spiritual balance in your life in order to stay healthy on all levels.

---

23 Learn more about Energy Psychology and the importance of clearing emotional blockages by going to: http://annemerkel.com/energy-psychology/

Point #13 - Structural Balance

If your body tissue is torqued or twisted, or your skeletal structure is misaligned, then your imbalance will probably cause pain at the very least, but more importantly, it may impede your physical functions. There are times when energy is blocked, muscles are "turned off", energy meridians are running too strong or too weak, tendons or ligaments are stretched or strained, and the body cannot function in a healthy fashion. There are experts who can help.

In my own experience, after falling off of my horse at age 17, I was told by a surgeon that I would have to wear a back brace for my entire life and never participate in athletics again. I lived for a few years in pain and worry with this prognosis, until I was introduced to my first chiropractic adjustment. Finding a practitioner whose practice was based solely on supporting health through structural balance solved my problems and helped me to create the active life that I desired.

I highly endorse Chiropractors or Osteopaths with diplomates in Manipulation, who have studied Applied Kinesiology or Clinical Kinesiology, both advanced techniques which allow the body to provide the practitioner the information about what it needs and how to fix it. These practitioners know how to turn muscles back on, balance meridians, check for allergens or nutritional deficits, and identify toxins. Structural balance is so important in its physical and energetic support of all the other systems in the body. Pay attention to it and use the appropriate practitioners in your structural maintenance.[24]

Point #14 - External Influences

I touched on that a little bit when I talked about the hygiene. External influences have to do with looking at toxins in your environment such as the cleaning agents that are used in your home, air fresheners, remodeling construction materials, glues, paints, out-gasses from new carpets or other materials, plus so many more things that you need to take the time to notice.

---

24 Here is a strong message about this from an Osteopathic physician: http://functionalforum.com/are-we-mistreating-structural-issues-with-biochemical-solutions/

If you have any of plug-in air filters that are supposed to make your room smell happy and fresh, unplug them and throw them in the garbage can now. Those things are poisonous and detrimental to your health. Any fake fragrances or phalates that are not natural essential oils, are artificial and can create a long list of negative symptoms. The artificial scent industry is a multi-billion-dollar industry worldwide, but it produces poisonous chemicals and you don't need to breathe their fake smells. If you want to infuse your surroundings with a good aroma, buy a high-grade essential oil. Choose the oil with which you relate based on both the odor and the energetic properties. Whatever you breathe goes right into your lungs and will help shift your energy as well as your mood – for the good or not so good, so choose well that which you breathe.

Here is what one of my clients, Lisa, said about her experience after I shared this information with her:

> "It was one simple thing but I feel that it was definitely life changing. Briefly, my mother and I share the same home. She had an automatic air freshener in her bedroom. It was set to operate around the clock, 24/7. It probably sprayed out maybe every 15 or 20 minutes. We didn't think much of it, even though we do have some other air fresheners that are all natural using just the orange oil, but they don't fit that little automatic machine. After a couple weeks, I started having flu-like symptoms and even missed some days of work. For me it was foggy head, general fogginess, headaches – I'm not a person that has headaches very often at all – digestive problems and a lot of nausea. I just couldn't figure out what it was. My mom kept saying that she felt very fatigued. She would come out of her room and say she was just so tired that she wanted to go back to bed.
>
> After hearing the great things you said, I still didn't speak to my mom. It took me about two days. One morning I said, 'Mom, if you could, let's turn this off and see if this may be our issue.' She turned it off around 1:00. By 6:00 that evening, we were both feeling better – it was very, very noticeable. We were really anesthetizing ourselves. That had gone on for about a month. We were really in bad

condition. I just want to thank you so much, Dr. Merkel. It was lifesaving. She would have just kept replacing those little spray bottles."

What we're talking about is the fact that our olfactory sense is hotwired right into the brain. It doesn't go through any other channels. It goes straight into the brain, so whatever you smell gives you an automatic impulse or some automatic reaction. When we're out in society, there are so many manmade chemical odors. Some of them are considered fragrances, some are perfumes, some are body lotion fragrances, some are considered hygienic and placed on sanitary napkins, adult diapers, and even in deodorants. If they're manmade, they could potentially be dangerous for your body. The only things that are really beneficial to the body would be the pure essential oils. Even then, you have to be careful because so many people have sensitivity to <u>any</u> odors.

Please be aware of what you have in your home and what you wear or carry with you; whatever you use in the way of fragrances. Be careful of everything you use, all the cleaners in your house, for your body, for your home, for your clothes, for your dishes. Don't buy any brands that have artificial odors. Those may really hurt you. If you need an odor to change what your inner room smells like, go to essential oils and choose some good, high-powered – not the cheap ones –true, pure essential oil. You can't get those in a drug store or a supermarket. Even potpourris so often have artificial things sprayed on them so that they smell good. You don't need any of that, so be a wise and healthy consumer!

Point #15 – EMF's

I need to throw in here how important it is to turn off and get away from Electro-Magnetic Frequencies (EMF's) – especially at night when you intend to sleep. I believe, just my hypothesis, that if you are sitting right next to your modem or Wi-Fi, or if you're constantly being zapped by your cell phone, TV, computer, tablet, iPod, iPad, your lymph is going to suffer and thicken into a slow-moving sludge. That's the way my body feels when I've spent too many hours in front of a computer and I haven't drunk enough water. You've got to drink even more water when you're around those devices. There are various helpful sources which will give you more scientific data about the dangers of EMF's.[25]

Point #16 – Grounding into the Earth

And, as a final point in this section, I highly endorse the whole concept of "earthing". It's so important to just go out barefooted and stand in the earth. That's not saying to walk without shoes on asphalt or most concrete because there are fillers and polymers that block the natural electro-magnetics of the earth. It will lessen your pain to be in touch with the earth's natural electro-magnetics and the electrons that it emits. I highly endorse this to anybody who has any chronic pain like fibromyalgia or even rheumatoid arthritis or basic arthritis. Don't walk on hard surfaces because that's not going to help your pain, but instead, go out and stand or sit and touch the ground. If there is a lot of grass, dig yourself a little hole and put your bare feet so that you're actually touching the earth. You will feel a difference. Sit out there 15 to 20 minutes. I guarantee that this will help. While you're doing that, move some muscles around, even if you're just walking in place or walking in a circle on gentle grass. That will make a big difference in how you feel. The earth can help you heal. Nature can help you heal. The electro-magnetics are naturally very healing. When we wear shoes with soles, we're blocking these. When we're walking on hard surfaces that are manmade, we are blocking these too. It is time to get back in touch with our home planet Earth so we can naturally re-balance.[26]

Point #17 - It's up to you! Attitude makes a difference!

Are you willing to put yourself as number one in your life? Your attitude is of utmost importance to your health, and I hope you realize by now that nobody else is going to put you as number one

---

25 See: Green, Debra. (2010) www.RadiationPage.com "Electromagnetic Frequencies (EMF) and Your Health" via http://YourEnergyMatters.com - and - Gittleman, Ann Louise. (2014) *Zapped: Why Your Cell Phone Shouldn't Be Your Alarm Clock and 1,268 Ways to Outsmart the Hazards of Electronic Pollution.* New York, NY: Harper Collins Publishers.
26 Learn about this concept and how you can re-connect directly or via "earthing products" by going to: www.earthinginstitute.net or read: Ober, Clinton; Sinatra, Stephen T., M.D.; Zucker, Martin. (2010) *Earthing: The most important health discovery ever?* Laguna Beach, CA:; Basic Health Publications, Inc. www.basichealthpub.com

except yourself. Your doctor is not going to put you as number one. It's up to you. The question to ask yourself is: "Will I put myself as number one?"

Ask yourself and write down answers to the following:

- Will I commit to drinking enough water?
- Will I change my diet?
- Will I get rid of the Teflon pans and aluminum cookware and use healthy cookware that's not leeching plastics or metals into my food?
- Will I stop eating the refined foods?
- Will I stop eating the gluten and things that can lead to worse autoimmune conditions?
- Am I ready to do that?
- Will I put myself first on the schedule for getting a full night's sleep and then let everything else come together?
- Will I put myself and my exercise as a high priority in my daily schedule?"

These questions are so important for you to ask of yourself in order to move forward to health. And, if you are feeling any level of resistance to the points I've mentioned here, you may use energy therapy meridian tapping to clear the resistance so you will be more open to making up your mind as to what you choose to undertake for the benefit of your own health.

It really is up to you!

My Energy Psychology Practice

Utilizing Energy Psychology with autoimmune disorders is merely one of many approaches that all kinds of physicians use. My approach is via the emotional component, which I find is regularly part of the autoimmune condition ratio. I utilize many different techniques, and several that I include in this book involve the connection with the client's energy meridians.

The practice of meridian tapping or holding has been used by numerous cultures world-wide for thousands of years. The human body is naturally nurtured when specific points along the energy channels are touched or enervated. The channels are referred to as meridians.

Meridians and Tapping Points

Meridians are pathways of energy making up the meridian system comprised of acupressure vessels located throughout the body. These contain a free-flowing colorless, non-cellular liquid which may be partly actuated by the heart. Meridians have been measured and mapped by modern technological methods, electronically, thermatically, and radioactively.

The electromagnetic points that we tap along the meridians are known as acupuncture points, and consist of small oval cells called Bonham corpuscles which surround the capillaries in the skin, the blood vessels, and the organs throughout the body.

There are 14 meridians in the body and in using EFT/ Emotional Freedom Techniques we utilize most of these in a simplified focus by tapping on a single point for each meridian. These are mainly the "end points" on the meridians that are tapped or other significant acupuncture points along specific meridians.

EFT / Emotional Freedom Techniques and NET / Neuro Emotional Technique

To date, I have been formally studying and utilizing various energy therapy tools for over thirty years. In the early 1980's I studied a variety of more esoteric modalities focused on frequency, including colors, sounds, crystals, hands-on healing, psychic phenomena, and channeling. In 1986 I was introduced to Applied Kinesiology in a class for chiropractors, and this paved the way for me to eventually become a practitioner of energy therapy with clients. During the early to mid-1990's I studied NET/ Neuro Emotional Technique[27] with various doctors and other licensed health practitioners. I slipped in with my Ph.D. and fell in love with how this technique allowed me to ask a client's body via muscle testing whether an issue was emotional, nutritional, chemical/ toxin-related, or structural. At the time I was studying I was already utilizing flower essences with clients and NET utilizes specially formulated homeopathics to assist in clearing "body memory" for clients with deep, long-standing emotional traumas. In the late 1990's I worked on my certification in Healing Touch, when through the initiations to become a Reiki Master, and while looking for a modality similar to NET that I could use on myself, I was introduced to EFT/ Emotional Freedom Techniques.[28] With this easy-to-learn and easy-to-apply/teach technique I was able to take my practice world-wide via the telephone, whereas using NET by itself requires me to work face-to-face with a client so I can do the meridian tapping along the client's spine after I've ascertained what the client needs via manual muscle testing. With all the background that I had learned in NET, combined with the ease of this new seeming "short-cut" method, EFT, I was armed with all that I needed to set out to help people.

You may access a free Introduction to EFT package where you will be guided as to how to use EFT the way I teach it, and there is a video demonstrating the specific tapping points, which meridians they enervate, and the emotions that 90% of the time are related to each meridian.[29]

The Use of Energy Therapy is Coming of Age

In the five years since I worked with Gerry, the first case mentioned in this book, my own approach to clients, and autoimmune in particular, has become much more thorough and in-depth because of my added years of experience plus diligent research and study of specialized tapping, applied kinesiology, energy medicine, and

---

[27] Visit www.netmindbody.com for more information.
[28] Learn more at: www.emofree.com
[29] Learn to use EFT at: www.annemerkel.com/free-eft-stuff

naturopathy. I don't include in this book the utilization of homeopathy, flower essences, essential oils, or other naturopathic approaches to clearing the emotional component from the "body memory". This will be included in my next book.

So many more tools and techniques are being accepted into main-stream western functional medicine, and people are turning to "alternative" tools because what has been offered through more traditional western systems simply does not work for everyone and for every case.

Since 2012 I have been training and Certifying coaches, therapists, physicians, and other health & wellness practitioners[30] in order for them to use a variety of energy therapy tools in their on-going practices.

There is now scientific evidence of the efficacy of utilizing these tools to clear emotional stress, and proof of the benefits of doing this as part of any other health protocol. Energy psychology modalities have been researched by more than 100 investigators in at least 7 countries. As of 2014, over 60 research studies have been published on specific modalities where only one has not shown efficacy.[31] And, this is just the tip of the iceberg, since there are many researchers and practitioners outside of the Energy Psychology arena who are also researching many of the same modalities and their effectiveness.

We are living in exciting times, and I feel like I am riding the wave into a new way of practicing health support. There is so much to learn about the implications of the mind and emotions on physical, mental, emotional, and spiritual health, and now the world is just awaiting practitioners who can support their healing. I feel blessed!

---

[30] Learn more: http://annemerkel.com/energy-therapy-certification/
[31] Although there are many other studies from other disciplines that utilize energy therapy modalities, and I will touch on more in my next book, go here to access the specific studies of Energy Psychology: http://www.energypsych.org/?Research_Landing

Autoimmune Cases

Case studies of any type include both the subjective and objective data, and in this book all of the clients met with me by telephone so there are recordings of certain aspects of the case. Auditory accounts can be quite revealing and in some of these cases the client was coached on a live group call, so there are instructions for those in the "audience" who wish to work along with the person on the "coaching seat".

If you read a case here and can relate to the symptoms or diagnosed condition or issues that we address, you may wish to contact me directly to ascertain whether there is a specific recording available that you may use as a support tool for your own case.[32]

I regularly work with clients in my **Autoimmune Coaching & Energy Therapy Support** call series. This series is now in its third year and still going strong with hundreds of participants registered and either participating on the live calls or enjoying the follow-up call recordings. You may register for this free series[33] or contact me directly to identify and receive a copy of a specific recording with which you relate.

By participating along with the audio recording you will automatically receive the "Borrowed Benefits" often discussed by EFT creator, Gary Craig.[34] I highly recommend that if you are suffering from any chronic ailment or autoimmune issue, that you consider joining the free call series... especially if you relate to anything that you read in the following cases.

And, if you are new to meridian tapping, I offer a free **Introduction to EFT Package** that you may access from one of my websites.[35]

For the purposes of this book reviewing cases of real Autoimmune clients and demonstrating how I worked in a session or over time

---

32 Contact me at: info@arielagroup.com
33 Register at: http://www.myeftcoach.com/autoimmune-coaching-support-group
34 For more information go to: http://emofree.com
35 Go to: http://arielagroup.com/products/free_products.php

with them, I try to cover some major themes and issues that I often find as background "causes" or contributing factors in these people developing conditions where the body works against itself. The specific conditions, symptoms, or themes that are highlighted in the specific cases that I have chosen are highlighted in the next **Overview of Cases** section.

In my next book I will touch on research that has been done linking certain personality "types" and behavior patterns such as some listed above, with the potential for developing autoimmune disorders. I'll also review some of the Naturopathic modalities that can be utilized effectively in working with the personal profiles as well as the physical symptoms to clear emotional residue or other energetic causes or components of the autoimmune disorders. More research is coming to light every day - and is originating from a variety of disciplines, so stay tuned!

Also, check back regularly to my website for new publications, research, presentation outlines and recordings from webinars, conference presentations, and other informative resources about autoimmune.[36]

---

36 Go to: http://annemerkel.com/autoimmune-programs .

Overview of Cases

My own case covered issues of dependence & independence related to my marriage and old belief system. The underlying struggle that went on, plus an imbalanced diet, led to a rough bout with **CFS/ Chronic Fatigue Syndrome** and **Fibromyalgia** with which I suffered for over a year. My symptoms included constant fatigue, fuzzy mind, loss of memory, horrible joint pain, and finally hair loss. I look back now and realize that although I feel that I wasted a year of my life being unhealthy and seemingly "useless" in my life, that year was a time of great learning that has helped me to serve others with autoimmune disorders.

Gerry's case was pivotal in my practice, and I intended from the beginning to write about her eventually. In her section I cover a full spectrum of issues that eventually led to her inability to show up in today's world as we know it. With **MCS/ Multiple Chemical Sensitivities** and body-wide **Psoriasis**, Gerry wore a carbon filter mask and generally stayed in her borrowed single bedroom most of the time until we connected. Her early life abandonment, abuse, and then life-long feelings of guilt led to her inner build-up of toxins which eventually was overloaded with a toxic chemical event in her place of work. She lived with constant weakness, fatigue, and flu-like symptoms based on her environment and rate of activity. Over several months we took every aspect of her life and used meridian tapping along with other energy therapy tools to unwind her emotional stressors so that she could be free to re-balance in health... which she eventually did!

Tanya's condition was **Graves Disease** (a **Hyper-thyroid** condition), and although she did not have the bulging eyes often associated with this malady, she did suffer with anxiety, joint pain, deep fatigue, & intestinal upset. Tanya's critical voice kept reminding herself that she didn't deserve to receive special treatment and that she should not be making a big fuss about herself. She had always subconsciously felt like a burden, so had many layers to dissolve in her re-balancing process toward health.

In **Sally's** case dealing with **CFS/ Chronic Fatigue Syndrome** and **Fibromyalgia**, the main theme of her life was that of a "Caretaker" for everyone other than herself. She had to learn to put her needs first in order to get well and then be able to take care of others in the quality ways she desired. With a full list of physical symptoms and an extensive list of negative emotions bogging her down, we had our work cut out for us. After working together for three months, or a total of nine hour-long phone sessions, Sally was ready to move forward in her life with a personal relationship that was triggering some of the old symptoms and fatigue. During the session shared in this book we supported Sally to realize her role in any relationship had to be first with herself, and then with others. To this day Sally's life and health continue to improve, and she is currently working with a specialist to clear the harmful effects of mold and mildew in her environment related to her health.

Amanda presents a very serious condition in her case: **Wegener's Vasculitis**, in which the body's blood flow gets cut off from major organs. Amanda had almost died and had spent extensive time in the hospital, part of which was in an induced coma. She came to me first with fear that her symptoms were returning and then later we worked together to help her lose the weight that she had taken on while on extensive steroid therapy. Amanda is a "poster child" for successful use of energy therapy tools, and she continues to improve to this day.

Amanda's case is an extreme example of how one's lifestyle and life stresses can start to kill a person. When Amanda first approached me she described her health and situation saying the following:

"In my early twenties I was covered in hives for over a year for no apparent reason. I think I had more hives at a later time for a couple of years. During the year before the major symptoms started I was extremely stressed out. I had quit smoking a few months before the skin blisters showed up. I have a difficult relationship with my mother where I am the parent, and from an early age I absorbed all of her problems and emotional stress. My father is also very difficult. I was starting to gain weight and had chronic throat infections. My son was two years old at the time and I am also guardian of my handicapped brother. Work was stressful and I lost a promotion because of being sick so much. I was also in part-time school working toward a degree. I also had a miscarriage six months prior. Just before I was hospitalized I got a new job."

If the above reminds you of your own story, then I advise that you run to your nearest Energy Psychologist to clear old behavioral patterns and stored emotional stress before your body shuts down. In Amanda's case she had ignored or masked early symptoms from her early 20's and later at age 30 her body started to shut down. Here is what she said about her lifestyle:

"I am a perfectionist and grew up thriving on crisis after crisis. I am working on not being like that and eliminating stress from my body. But, I think my past is keeping me sick still. During my entire recovery I have continued to go to school for my degree. I believe this too has had an impact on my health. I am in my last two courses and will be returning to work when I finish. I just want to be well for myself, husband, and son." Even in her sickest time Amanda was still driving herself. This is a good example for all *Type A Personalities*, who have a tendency for the later development of autoimmune disorders,[37]or even *Highly Sensitive* or empathic people who also have a propensity for taking on stresses leading eventually to autoimmune in some individuals.[38]

Veronica suffered from hyper vigilance from a violent father, and her condition of never being able to speak her truth during much of her life eventually led to the autoimmune thyroid condition, Hashimotos Thyroiditis.

Helen similarly suffered from a controlling father and absent mother and was split between two countries. Because of the loss and the control exerted over her by one or both parents, she presented with lung ailments – asthma from the feelings of loss, and skin ailments – eczema, psoriasis, hives from both loss and feeling like a victim of control by others... both of these considered "metal" element meridian energetics.

---

37 See: Leary, Mark, Ph.D. (2012). **Understanding the Mysteries of Human Behavior: Course Guidebook & Audio.** Chantilly, VA: The Great Courses Publishers

38 Sodi, Carla M. (2015) "PART 1: The Bond Between Autoimmune Diseases and Highly Sensitive Persons" **– The Tapping Solution Website.** April 13, 2015. " PART 2: The Hidden Link Between Highly Sensitive People and Autoimmune Disorders" **– The Tapping Solution Website.** April 20, 2015. http://www.thetappingsolution.com/eft-articles/category/carla-m-sodi

This and the last case are both similar and different, representing different women from different cultures and different age groups, and yet both presented with somewhat similar skin-related symptoms which responded well to energy therapy meridian tapping.

Kristen's case, like the previous one, also involved a strong sense of loss – of love, of her father, of her mother's love, of her life security. We worked together to clear various issues involved and her skin started to clear up.[39]

Then, surprising even to Kristen, herself, as she became stronger in self love and self-esteem, she made some life-changing decisions that caused stress in her life as she began to implement the steps toward the new directions she chose. She came back to me for a session to help her clear the fear of moving forward. This is somewhat similar to Amanda's follow-up session, however in Kristen's case, she was older and in a different stage of life, and she was initiating some de-stressing moves as she began to simplify her life for better health and quality.

Kristen's case is different in some ways than others because of a possible deeper grade trauma stress that happened during a plane crash when she was 17 years old. I've included some pertinent information about Stephen Porges' Polyvagal Theory which I believe has led to genetic mutations and caused Kristen to experience a Near-Death episode during the plane crash. This can definitely leave a body-mind-spirit somewhat altered... and, the good news is that, according to Porges, energy psychology can support the re-balancing and healing of even these kinds of deep physiology-psychology experiences.

---

[39] See the dramatic "before" and "after" photos of Kristen's legs in her case chapter.

Gerry

When I started working with Gerry on March 23 of 2010, I recognized a kindred spirit. She had signed up for an energy therapy coaching session with me, and I realized from the beginning that there was a special being struggling to speak from her very weakened and vulnerable body.

She shared that for thirteen years she had suffered from **MCS/ Multiple Chemical Sensitivity** syndrome[40], or "environmental illness", which is considered an autoimmune disorder because it creates an inner "allergy" to life in general. By the time I met her, Gerry had lost everything she owned, had spent most of a year, including a hard northeastern winter, living in her car when her friend's cabin was occupied, and now stayed in another friend's upstairs bedroom where she slept on a mattress on the floor and managed to pull herself across the floor and up to a counter where she cooked on a single hotplate. When she went outside she had to wear a breathing mask so that the fragrances, pollen, environmental odors would not literally knock her out. She also battled psoriasis over most of her emaciated and weakened body.

I suggested that we work together because I was most interested in her case. After about five weeks, she sent me a picture showing that she had improved so much that she had the stamina and inner strength to go out in public again without wearing a mask.

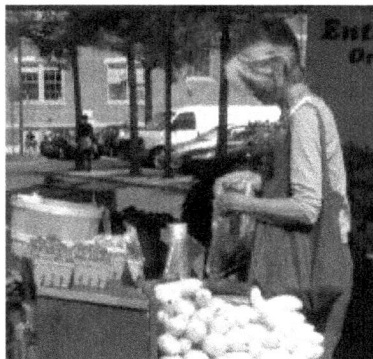

---

[40] See **Appendix 1** for more information about this condition.

Gerry's case and history represent several classic themes that show up often in autoimune conditions. I discovered the following:

- A climactic event triggered the collapse of her life and health after many years of emotional turmoil;
- Her early life included traumas of abandonment, strife between parents, physical abuse, shame & embarrassment;
- She grew up feeling out of control, unable to speak up for herself, helpless, hyper-vigilant of what trauma was coming next, and generally feeling pushed aside like a burden without worth.

The issues above represent a recipe for health disaster if a person doesn't catch the earlier symptoms in time, and in Gerry's case it took a major chemical exposure to trigger the eventual healing of emotional poisons that had been with her for 65 years.

Gerry's Story

In 1997 Gerry felt like she had it all: a good job as full-time Manager of a Fine Arts Center at a church, a nice condo that she bought herself, friends, volunteer projects, and the life she was building was moving forward from a difficult childhood and failed marriage with estranged children then in college. She was optimistic and started to see a positive future in her life – maybe for the first time.

At some point in 1997 the church decided to place a dance studio in the Arts Center and they placed mirrors all over the walls held on by high resin epoxy glue. Even though they used fans and vents after they hung the mirrors, the head teacher went home and vomited, and several other people in the office area had headaches. Gerry persevered and after three days of full-time work in that environment she was found unconscious at her desk.

They called the EMS who took her out and placed her on oxygen. She regained consciousness finally after almost an hour, and nobody fully realized how the traumatic event affected her brain. She reported that in the emergency room she felt like people were treating her like she was crazy, and this made her angry even though she was so debilitated that she couldn't do anything about it.

We later cleared this anger and the inability of the hospital staff to see her as a victim of poisoning to the brain.

Her first symptoms were running eyes, difficulty breathing, light headedness, and she noticed that anything in the environment started being totally bothersome to her: flowers, the pesticides in the fields around the town where she lived, any kind of environmental impact hurt her physical system. Other symptoms that Gerry had included eyes watering, brain on alert, immune and lymphatic reactions, and she felt drugged out with a lot of brain fog.

After about one month Gerry started working from home but then she realized she couldn't continue, and by that point she was so sick and weak that she couldn't even go back to say goodbye or clean out her desk. The people she worked with took up a collection for her because insurance was not committing to pay her very much, and the disability was limited. That was the end of Gerry's working career at the Art Center, and the beginning of a downward spiral.

Like so many others suffering from chronic, debilitating conditions – most classified under the heading of autoimmune, Gerry was working up to getting sick, and it took one accident to push her over the edge. As an Energy Psychologist "detective", I look into people's histories to discover the "last straw", and then I go back to identify the root causes of the stress leading up to that final break-down.

In Gerry's case, there were many things that set her up for later suffering.
- At a very young age Gerry felt the terror of being lost in a store, and it seemed to her that nobody cared to come looking for her.
- Out of her own issues, Gerry's mom deserted her family when Gerry was 5 years old, but then later returned.
- As a young child Gerry was physically and emotionally abused by her alcoholic mother who could be quite violent at times. Her father was there but did nothing to protect her. She grew to feel like she should be invisible or take up no space, so as to not bother or trigger anybody, and then be safe.
- She was a young child and had no "voice" in asking for what she needed or for fending off abuse.

- She felt like a burden and felt abandoned from constantly being left to wait for her mother, who was always late to appointments to pick her up.
- She felt personally accosted by anybody who made changes in her environment without her being a part of the decision, because she had no control in her early life with her parents and never knew what horrible thing was just around the corner.
- Later as a teen Gerry was humiliated by her mother's horrible psoriasis when she exposed her legs to Gerry's teenaged friends in public, and later developed psoriasis herself, which caused her to hate her body.[41]
- She felt ashamed, unworthy of love, lonely, and later guilty when she left her loving husband and two children. She didn't know how to be loved, even when it was directed at her. She didn't love herself because growing up she had no model for being loved. She had felt like a time bomb ready to go off, so like her mother had done before, Gerry left.
- At some time in her life she lost faith in God when she felt unprotected in a dire time of need. This left her feeling hopeless without faith that anyone cared. Later in our work she began again to feel her connection with her God, but it took lots of work to overcome her inner resistance to re-connecting with Source.

Gerry was brimming over with negative feelings from her past: anxiety, hyper-vigilance, victimhood, resignation, acceptance, anger, resentment, fear, abandonment, helplessness, hopelessness, shame, guilt, unworthiness, deceived, out-of-control, lack, loss & grief, among others. She was addicted to negative thinking and even though she was doing well outwardly in 1997, on the inside there were poisons brewing.

Our Work Together

As we began working together Gerry had just been introduced to

---

[41] Gerry probably inherited her mother's physical as well as emotional genetic predisposition to skin issues, plus the memories of staring at her mother's psoriasis lesions imprinted in her subconscious. Additional emotional issues of grief and loss triggered skin reactions which created that as her major organ for toxic elimination later in life.

EFT tapping and she participated in a week-long EFT Tapping series of calls on-line which she enjoyed. In developing her own "personal style" of tapping Gerry had special meridian tapping points that felt more comfortable to her, including:

- tapping the inside of her wrist,
- holding the left index finger like a handlebar then holding the right thumb with her left fingers, (so that she would create a kinesiology circuit holding both her lung and her large intestine meridians,)[42]
- she also would hold her in her wrists together, and
- she used the *Top of Her Head* points

There were several reasons why she used additional meridian points including:

- she had so much psoriasis all over her body that it was very difficult for her to tap on some of the traditional EFT tapping points,

and of even more significance in our work,

- she felt assaulted whenever she tapped on her face because of the traumatic abuse she had endured as a child at the hands of her mother. We worked together to clear the abuse.

When I worked in 2010 with Gerry by phone I used mainly EFT/ Emotional Freedom Techniques meridian tapping and some of the more spiritual and esoteric techniques involving bringing in deceased ancestors to clear issues toward forgiveness, "recreating the story" of past traumatic memories, neuro-lymphatic rubbing, neuro-vascular holding, among others. You will note that I go beyond this in my other cases which reflect work I did in 2014-15.

Gerry really grew to understand the potency of focusing on her feelings as she was tapping on the meridian points. At one point she put it bluntly: "Your stressing, 'Just tap, tap, tap . . . feeling the feeling and tapping without labeling,' is helpful." So it's not about

---

[42] By enervating both her lung and large intestine meridians at the same time she was supporting her "metal element meridians" which are most related to skin issues. Over the time we worked together the severity and patterns of the psoriasis on her body changed and started to abate.

the words you say when you're doing meridian tapping; it's about getting into the feelings of the memory or issue, and clearing the emotional charge.

While I was working with the emotional components of Gerry's case, she was following a diet recommended by a local naturopath which included herbal teas, and she used specialized homeopathics. She practiced Qigong daily whenever she was able. I was happy to be helping with the emotional component while Gerry relied on others to support her body's rebalancing.

Although Gerry's personality was one of a leader, survivor, assertive intelligent person, because of her abusive background she felt like a victim – which made her mad. And, there was a part of her that didn't feel that she "deserved to heal". I find this subconscious blockage in many chronically or critically ill people, and the key is to identify the original point at which the person started to feel "unworthy to exist", and when that is cleared, the reluctance to heal usually collapses also.

Gerry also had a severe inner critical voice that constantly reprimanded and berated her before she began to use meridian tapping on a daily basis. This inner negativity reflected an inner sense of deficiency in herself, and we worked on this coming from many directions, clearing as many aspects as showed up.

She related to me how she had experienced difficulties as a child learning to read, and her mother used the strap on her when she made mistakes. Even when she wasn't doing badly the strap sat with them as she and her mother went over her reading lessons. Gerry went on to earn an MS degree in psychiatric nursing. This early abuse easily led to many years of anxiety and hyper-vigilance which caused great stress in Gerry's system.

During the first month or so that we worked together I noticed an aggressive and almost belligerent attitude from Gerry whenever I had to re-schedule a session or if I were a minute late to our session having just left working with another client. I managed to fit Gerry into my busy schedule as a favor to her, however because of her past pattern of abuse, neglect, lack of respect, and feelings of abandonment, she was almost abusive to me as her caregiver.

This sometimes happens in cases of people who have suffered chronic illness and great personal loss. They may lash out at those closest to them in imbalanced manners reflecting their inner anguish and old patterns of emotional hurt. Each time this happened I walked Gerry through it and helped her to focus on the real source of her agitation, so she could work the causes out and clear the local agitation with me at the same time.

Starting to see Results

Following our session on April 16, just two and a half weeks after her first session, Gerry reported:

> "Noticeable sense of energy and well being- went outside and walked to store a block away which I hadn't done in several weeks. Afterwards walked at the park and took in the glorious day and blooming flowering trees and sky and earth and am filled with joy and gratitude. Then had dinner at my friend's house with her two kids- really nice to be out and about.
>
> I chose not to dwell on our session and I don't plan to listen right away to the tape of today as the releasing was profound and I don't feel going back into that space is useful."

Gerry, like many people suffering from autoimmune disorders, was very sensitive to EMF/ electro-magnetic frequencies, so she tried to stay away from using her computer or any other device as much as possible. Her pre- and post-coaching reports were always short and to the point without regard to grammar.

During the April 15 session we had focused on clearing resentment, a sense of not deserving, and the psoriasis. We tapped on issues related to her mother's chronic and almost intentional tardiness creating more abandonment issues in Gerry. We also addressed victimhood, and I had her pretend she was a little girl talking to her mother, and she was able to finally speak about her feelings to her mom as a child, letting out lots of stuffed emotion. It was a potent session with good results as reflected in her comments.

During Gerry's session on April 22nd we worked on her mother issues around victimhood, deception, abandonment, and feeling out of control. She was able to speak her anger and disappointment, and reported the following:

> "After our session, I rested- took a nap and was with the healing. Then I took a baking soda detox bath which became a ritual cleansing of victimhood. I ended the bath with a cold shower to release and step forward free from that vibration.
>
> I feel a new connection with Ma including inviting her guides (I remember her speaking to them as a teenager and I hated it) to join us in this healing adventure. I caringly applied cream to my skin with Ma in mind as if I was soothing her skin as well (I NEVER imagined I would imagine doing that!). I also offered this healing to all beings especially those with psoriasis.
>
> Then, I cooked a delicious nutritious meal to nourish this healing body of mine and ate outside. I noticed as I walk, I stand tall and feel regal (the opposite of victim for sure!). I went for over an hour walking in nature and taking in the beauty of sky, earth, and bird sounds.
> Home now, I've just completed another round of qigong which I do each morning now to a DVD."

Like Gerry, her mother had suffered inner and outer traumas in life and these reflected in how she parented Gerry, the subconscious imprints she left on her daughter, as well as the DNA that she shared with her offspring. Her mother was in the Philippines during the world war and almost died young of malaria. She more-than-likely lived a life of anxious hyper-vigilance and possibly carried hopeless victimhood into her marriage and motherhood. Different "mother issues" come up during our work together and we cleared them one-by-one.

A very profound session took place after I asked Gerry to fill in the **Personal Values Assessment** exercise.[43] When she did this I realized that she had placed her health as #5 in priority out of 10 items. This showed me that she still had a block to healing with

---

[43] Sign up for this at: www.annemerkel.com/eft-free-stuff

some inner belief that it was not appropriate, important, she was not worthy, nobody wanted her to be healthy and happy, etc. She even believed that God wanted her to stay sick, so she was debilitated in being able to commit and choose health as a priority.

During two sequential sessions we:
1- focused on allowing Gerry to feel open to healing,[44] and then
2- cleared the old feelings of unworthiness and her inability to truly love and accept herself.[45]

In our last wrap-up session Gerry commented on how potent those sessions' results had been when she said:

> "The values assessment presented a big 'aha!' for me. That's what my focus had been in these years since the toxic event: wanting to get healthy. To realize that, (she had placed her health as #5) really made a radical shift in how I perceived what I did each day. Sensing, 'Wait a minute, is this in alignment with the value that's highest in my priorities right now?' That was really pretty amazing to think that I could be thinking 'I'm working on my health,' and realize actually…. What really stood out was getting help wasn't my first priority. When I made that switch, I felt a shift in energies and alignments and intention. So, starting from that place, I remember a shift of what was possible."

In her summary of working with me she also stated:

> "I think one of the tapping sessions that stands out, among a couple that stand out, is the tapping session after which I stopped scratching the psoriasis with the kind of self-hate I had been doing up till that time. I always knew it was driven by something. I remember listening to that tape more than once, probably three or four times. I think it was three or

---

[44]To give you a glimpse of what we covered in this session and others with extensive meridian tapping sequences, I have included a section at the end of this book with **Tapping Sequences**. You may find Gerry's session tapping transcript for this issue listed as **Tapping Sequence 1**.
[45] For this issue see **Tapping Sequence 2**.

four weeks that I didn't scratch at all, which had not happened in 13 years.

Although that has returned, it no longer is with the intensity that I cannot stop. That piece dissolved and has not returned. That's major. Whatever else is going on with the psoriasis, the skin still does its thing. I've come more to 'this is how it is', not with so much resignation as a victim, but accepting that the skin is a detox organ. At some point, I like to think there will be a way that I can cleanse my body. It's clear to me that recently when I recorded 27 times in one hour that I had negative thought patterns, I'm still doing the detox from that mental-emotional level."

I'd like to share the tapping sequence(s) that we used during the session(s) on psoriasis that she refers to above.[46] Skin issues turn up regularly in autoimmune cases, and once the client or his/her practitioner looks deeper inside the skin, there are often specific reasons why the skin manifests the nasty sores and irritations. There are actually three significant tapping sequences that led up to a time when Gerry stopped scratching and the psoriasis started to heal. (We'll talk more about skin in Kristen's case.)

During the time we worked together I felt that there was a bond that formed, and even though Gerry is older than I am, I felt that she felt nurtured by my support as though I were a parent or close family member that showed up late in life. We talked things out together and she told me her deepest fears and embarrassments. Just like family members we pushed each other's buttons, and both grew together as Gerry's condition continued to improve.

During our final session Gerry remarked:

"I'd like to underline that being joined by you and having you kind of holding the space for the healing process that I was in, just like I said, was a gift from God, a gift from the

---

[46] Even though Gerry remembers this as one pivotal session, she actually had three sessions that together seemed to have supported her to stop itching and to regard the psoriasis skin condition more as a spectator than a victim. Each of these was different in the aspect that it focused to clear and the style of the session itself. See **Tapping Sequences 3 & 4 & 5.**

Universe. That was something. I felt really blessed by the time you spent and by learning the skill of tapping.

The tapping, which was new to me, opened up a doorway. What I liked about it, even though doing it together with you let me learn it in a very personal way, your process also let me learn on my own, particularly by having the recordings that I would listen to, and of just being able to go over again those places that felt most juicy. That way I could do a session over and over.

I felt, over time, I began to have the ability to create my own tapping scripts. Even now, I don't feel they're as full as I sense they are when we're on a Tapping Group call together or when I read some scripts. But, they're good enough to help me with a situation. They seem pretty simplistic in a certain way, yet just one of the lessons you taught me, and I guess it's because you said it so many times, taught me a lot. You said: 'Just tap the feeling. Just feel the feeling and let go of the words.' That was really useful. I understood what that meant. That had a meaning to me and I could work with that."

When asked what she felt was the most potent aspect of working together she said:

"I think the exposure. I thought that I was learning just the tapping and yet what I soon came to realize is how many tools you have in your 'toolbox.' The times we did guided meditation and calling in guides, I could feel the power of that on the session. It would stay with me. It's not something that I've been able to feel that I can acknowledge and access on my own. I may be accessing it, but I'm not able to feel that connection, even though it may well be happening. Having had those times together, where the power of it was more palpable, that's in there for me. I'm aware that it has registered and I can still feel it."

I feel that the above is not only a "thank you" to me, but also reflects what I hear from many clients who choose to work with a practitioner rather than "going it alone".

Final Words on Gerry's Case

After Gerry and I ended our time together we stayed in touch, and she still checks in with e-mails or shows up on group calls sometimes. She reported in 2012 that in addition to her EFT tapping practice, yoga, and qigong, she has learned another skill that she feels has helped her to re-program her thinking process about the MCS condition and her sensitivities to odors.

Ashok Gupta calls his specialized approach to clearing stress reactions to traumatic stimuli the *Gupta Amygdala Retraining Program*.[47] Using the program Gerry reports that now whenever she smells an odor or sees an unrecognizable liquid she can catch herself before she has a physiological reaction to the traumatic trigger. This ability to stop the automatic limbic brain reaction allows her to change her perception and expectations around odors and liquids, and to create new, healthier neural pathways allowing her to move toward health and living in the environment safely.

Before ending I want to share two other tapping sequences that I used in Gerry's sessions with great results. These also focused on changing her expectations before something she dreaded so that she had no extra stress or physical melt-down reactions.

One situation had to do with having a tooth extracted and her fears about the release of toxins into her body in addition to painful side effects that might all drain her fragile energies.[48]

The second situation was when she chose to drive to her daughter's home over three hours away. This was a long drive with the potential for heavy traffic and much stress, and the thought of it stretched her weakened physical and mental abilities to the limit. She ended up creating her own tapping protocol before and during her trip based on her experience with the dental extraction situation.

---

[47] You may learn more about his programs for MCS, Chronic Fatigue, Fibromyalgia, and more by going to:
http://www.guptaprogramme.com/mcs-multiple-chemical-sensitivity-treatment
[48] See **Tapping Sequence 6.**

In both cases Gerry's expectations of stress were enough to trigger a physical reaction, so in each case we cleared her expectations, changed her perceptions, and she flowed through both situations with flying colors and very little stress or pain. She later said:

> "I know when I was going to my daughter's at one point and had some apprehension on the drive because it was so far and my energy was so weak, just doing the tapping session and tapping in what it was going to be like to go there with a sense of ease of travel, while listening to a tape, and looking forward to seeing my grandchildren: that was one of the best driving trips I've had.

> I've used that imagery when I repeat the trip. Again, it's more the driving time. Rather than assuming it's a long trip and there's going to be traffic, it doesn't have to be that way.

> How I think it's going to be has a lot to do with it. It's the understanding that our beliefs and how the unconscious beliefs influence our behavior was a huge part of what I have learned from you, in a very vivid, concrete way. To me, being kinesthetic, being able to touch my body and being able to tap in ideas or tap out ideas is something I value deeply."

It was my honor to work with Gerry and to see her re-claim her life on so many levels!

-Tanya -

Tanya, like the other clients mentioned in subsequent cases, sent me a written history before we worked together on a live Autoimmune Support call. That gave me a lot of information.[49] She also took an on-line assessment instrument based on physical symptoms and their frequency.[50] This told me exactly what her meridians were doing so that I knew what priorities her body was proposing. Often we have something that we logically wish to work on, and we want instant results. If the body is not ready to let go of that particular issue because it has more layers around it that are a higher priority for the body, then it's not going to do what we consciously want it to do. That is why it's very important to make sure that I start to work with the body's first priority... otherwise a "fix" won't hold and I'll have to go back and address it again.

As I started out the call with Tanya I asked her to focus on the fact that for some reason her body was trying to tell her something - maybe that there was something in her that it needed to get rid of, something that was toxing it out to such an extent that it was starting to beat up on itself. Usually when that happens there's an emotional component. Why else would a body try to hurt itself? The body doesn't really know how to be sick. The body is a master at re-balancing, as long as its owner has stopped covering it up with toxins, which could be toxins of emotions, air, water, food, allergens, stressful situations, a bad environment, among other things. I told Tanya that this was a good opportunity for her to become a detective in her own life because only she knew what may be the basic causes for her body to be so confused and so upset that it actually was attacking itself. That's what happens with autoimmune.

At this point Tanya explained in her own words about her condition.

> "It feels complex. I have been diagnosed with Graves' disease. It's an autoimmune disease that attacks the thyroid and the eye tissues. My symptoms have been related to the thyroid primarily. It's under control. Blood test-wise it's

---

[49] See **Appendix 2**– Pre-coaching Intake Form
[50] Check out http://wellnesscheckonline.com .

been under control with medications for the past year.

I struggle with what I call generalized anxiety, kind of this constant sense of not doing enough, not being enough, not good enough. I've got some digestive symptoms. I have sort of random joint pain, just a lot of things that don't make sense. The thing that bothers me the most is just my emotional state. I have a hard time feeling present in my life. I feel like I don't control my life very well. I feel like I have low motivation. I'm very mentally fatigued. It's hard to focus, hard to concentrate. That's the thing that bothers me the most. My symptoms right now, wanting to do this live coaching call, and choosing to do this, is bringing up every voice inside me that says I don't need this, I don't deserve this. The physical sensations in my body right now are pretty significant. When you were describing being in the center of the circle, that's a trigger for me to feel like I shouldn't be there, that I'm making a big deal about this."

I next asked Tanya to start tapping on a set of points I call the **Heart Center**[51] while we continued to go over details from her history. This is often very helpful in that it starts to grab the attention of the limbic mind and viscera as well as the electro-magnetic biofield, and as emotions come up they are automatically addressed as the client is speaking of a historical event.

While Tanya tapped I asked her to focus on the following:

"It doesn't matter. You're making too big a thing out of this. It's not always that your GI tract is messed up. It's not always that you've got your joint pain and you're miserable with it. It's not always that you've got your low moods and high moods. Sometimes you do feel good. With Graves' disease in your particular case, Tanya, at least it's not

---

[51] For the **Heart Center**: You put your index finger in the middle of your upper chest, which is around where the thymus gland is located. If you're into chakras, it's your high heart chakra. Then put your middle finger right where a woman's cleavage begins and the other two fingers below that. You'll have your four fingers in a vertical line with three of them between your breasts and one of them higher than that in the middle of your upper chest.

bothering your eyes and you don't have bulging eyes like some people do. I just want you to scan yourself. Focus on any feelings of: I don't need this. I don't deserve this. I'm making too much of this. I shouldn't be here in the center. Why should I be here? Somebody else is probably sicker than I am. Any feelings like that, I want you to just feel those feelings."

I used words that came directly from Tanya's history report, so focusing on certain thinking patterns, I was helping to move into the deeper issues that might be holding the key to why Tanya was suffering from Graves' disease.

Quieting the Inner Critic

I next suggested that she focus on her "critical voice" to identify if that was her own voice or the voice of someone from her past or present. She was still tapping on the **Heart Center**.

"Whoever's voice comes up does not matter - you have lots of voices that speak in your own head. Sometimes it's your own voice that you've developed over the years; it's the critical voice. Sometimes it's a parent's voice or a doctor saying: 'Nothing showed up on your test so it's all in your head. Just go home and live with it. There's nothing we can do for it. You should be glad you're not as bad as some people.' That doesn't really make you feel any healthier.

Just breathe in a big breath of pure, healing energy. Feel it coming into your body and going to any of those feelings that you may have physically. Have it go to the unworthiness thoughts. Just imagine that this wonderful pure light and pure healing vibration has the ability to completely dissolve these thoughts and turn the volume down on those inner voices. Breathe out all the debris as it starts to loosen up. Start to let go of and mute that inner critical voice."

In most cases I like to remind people that they are always doing the best they can do in every moment and that it is the same for those around them. In Tanya's case I reminded her that she was human so was bound to have made mistakes in her life... and that people like doctors and her early care-givers also were human, so probably did not know everything needed to really help her in the ways that she always needed to be helped or guided.

Pregnancy and Birth Issues

Tanya was an unexpected pregnancy and the first child for her parents. They had not been together very long. Her mother had many fears, as do all first time moms – especially when they had not planned to get pregnant so early in the relationship. Some of the issues that we tapped on which she probably took on while she was in her mother's womb included:

- Fears about being a first-time mother,
  - ○ Pregnancy fears,
  - ○ Birth fears,
  - ○ "Will I be ready?" fears,
  - ○ "Will I be a good mom?" fears,
  - ○ "Will I have a supportive partner?"
  - ○ "Can we afford a baby?"
- Surprise or shock,
- Fears of what the father might think.

Because when we are in the womb we take on the vibrations of everything our mother feels, the fears above and the stress or uneasiness around these and other issues might cause an innate reaction of feeling like a burden or feeling like we are causing our mother pain, anguish, worry, and that makes us feel "bad"... and sometimes later undeserving of love.

We continued to tap on any subconscious fears about these issues. I heard lots of yawns in the coaching call audience indicating that there were energy shifts occurring in the people who were doing the energy therapy processes and tapping along with Tanya on their own issues. We were basically clearing universal issues that most people carry to some degree.

In Tanya's case, she felt like a burden and that she was not supposed to depend on others... because that "put them out".

Tanya's dad was a Vietnam vet with PTSD/ post traumatic stress disorder. He was very fragile. Maybe her mom wasn't quite ready to get pregnant with her until she was more confident and comfortable in the relationship. And, maybe her dad, even though he loved his wife and may have been open to having children, was shocked by the news of the pregnancy - as he was already emotionally brittle. There are many things that we don't know about any case, however there are always clues, and a good energy therapist detective holds the responsibility to look into all possibilities and tap away potential issues.

Anxiety

When Tanya was conceived her father already had PTSD; he had a lot of traumatic stuff in his psyche from war, and her mother reacted to his behavior in their relationship. We all inherit emotional traumas and psychological predispositions in our DNA from our parents, our grandparents, our great-grandparents. Any trauma that an ancestor has experienced before we're conceived comes into our own genes and, under the right stressful conditions, pops out unexpectedly.[52] We also take on modeled behaviors from our early care-givers. For Tanya this might have shown up as the anxiety she had felt most of her life. She admitted that she had suffered the stress of hyper vigilance all of her life where she was always on alert.

She started to understand in the session that her father in Vietnam had necessarily been hyper vigilant in order to stay alive. Her mother had to be alert to her father's moods and actions. She was starting to understand why she had felt so traumatized most of her life – without any real traumas of her own.

Anybody with post traumatic stress is always looking for what's going to attack them. They've been traumatized in one way or another. The triple warmer meridian is triggering the secretion of so many stress hormones at all times, that the only way they can tune it down is to drug themselves or to be drugged. Many veterans do that, just in order to calm down and to not feel the constant stress of: "Where's the next guerilla? Where's the next ambush? Where's the next attack going to come from?" It seemed that Tanya did not inherit being in the war, but she did inherit the

---

[52] For better understanding you may refer to: Church, Dawson, PhD. (2007) *The Genie in Your Genes: Epigenetic Medicine and the New Biology of Intention.* Santa Rosa, CA: Elite Books.

automatic subconscious stress responses from her father as well as the behavioral tendencies of her mom.

As we continued to tap, I asked Tanya to think back in her own life to the first time she consciously knew she was feeling anxious. I wanted to know if there was something that happened that had triggered a stress level that would then bring up the genetic predisposition to anxiety that she had inherited from her dad. She responded with the following:

> "The memories I have of being really anxious had to do with disappointing my father or feeling like he was not going to love me or he was going to leave. I have some specific memories of times when he was, I call it, 'having a temper tantrum', and that would be when I felt like I needed to fix it, I needed to behave better. Then to me it was constantly reinforced that I was supposed to make sure I didn't make dad mad because he would leave and he wouldn't love us or love me. That's what my hypervigilance was about, it seemed like, just constantly being aware of his emotions and walking on eggshells. Don't talk, don't feel."

We moved the meridian tapping to the EFT **Collar bone Point**.[53] Our focus was the fear that "little Tanya" might have felt whenever her father was around... that fear of upsetting him to the point that he would have one of his "tantrums" and leave her forever.

We also tapped away the results of the fear – the fact that "little Tanya" had to always be on her best behavior so that he wouldn't get upset, meaning that she couldn't be herself. She was never free and actually disappeared into the anxious being that she became. Tanya was never able to be a happy little girl running around and having a good time. Instead she was taking care of her father's emotional state and needed to stay on her guard around him or else

---

[53] Note that when I work with a client I have them tap continually on specific meridian points as we discuss or go over a variety of issues. As the emotions shift around the issues we change the location of tapping. This is the technique that I call N-hanced EFT, or the combination of NET/ Neuro Emotional Technique plus EFT/ Emotional Freedom Techniques. You may learn more about the specific tapping points by going to: http://annemerkel.com/free-eft-stuff/

keep away from him altogether.

I asked her to think about the time when her dad locked himself in a room for two days and Tanya was at the door trying to get him to come out and he refused to come out. I asked if she still had any level of emotional charge on that memory - based on a scale of zero to ten, with zero being no charge and ten being still very emotional.

Tanya responded that she still held about an 8-9 charge on that scale, and the event had happened when she was 7 years old.

I asked her to focus on the following:

> "You were young and he was in there. He was separating himself from you and the others. He wouldn't come out. Maybe that was a good thing for him with post traumatic stress when he was out of balance, to hide himself. However, to you, it was abandonment. I want you to go into that feeling of: 'Daddy won't come out. Daddy doesn't love me. Daddy won't talk to me. Is he really in the room? Is he ever going to come out? Is he okay? Is he hurting himself? Is he going out the window on the other side and I don't even know it? Have I lost him? Is he mad? Why is he in there? What did I do wrong? I must have done something wrong or else he wouldn't have locked himself in there.' At that age it's always our fault, even though it's not, but we think it is when an adult acts in a strange way that we can't understand. Just go into memories like that. Go in and feel that. Little Tanya is sitting outside that door trying to get her daddy to answer her, to come to the door. Do you feel that in your body anywhere?"

Tanya responded that she felt a sensation in her throat and upper chest. I continued:

> "While you're continuing to tap there on the **Collarbone Points**, I want you to put your other hand right at your throat.[54] Let's go back to that memory. You are the adult

---

54 This is a classic case of a young person being stifled in her ability to state her "truth". For so many years Tanya had bottled up her emotions, and the energy of the throat energy vortex or chakra had been blocked. This is seen

Tanya. Go back there to be with that little girl Tanya. You're going to be her spokesperson. You will tell your dad what little Tanya maybe really wanted to tell dad but was unable at the time. You're going to talk to him as an adult. What would you like to tell your father outside that door? Do you have anything you'd like to share?"

Tanya stated:

"I really hate when you have temper tantrums. It makes me feel like I'm not loved and that I can't depend on you to be there for me."

Then as the perpetual caregiver to her dad, Tanya stated:

"I just want to tell you that we're okay and you can come out."

At this point the sensation in Tanya's throat seemed to lessen. I asked her to put **one hand at her throat and the other hand across her forehead**.[55] At the same time I asked her to go into that feeling in her throat to feel the energy there and to breathe it out. I directed her to feel the sensation and to follow it if it moved from the throat to another location, to move the hand from the throat to wherever the sensation went while leaving the other hand across the forehead. I asked her to focus on the sensation and to breathe it out until she felt a shift.

"Think back to being outside that door and having your dad lock himself inside for two days and how you felt. Just breathe out those emotions. Just let them go now. You've been carrying them long enough. Breathe it out. He's locked himself in there. You're afraid for him. You feel abandoned. You feel that he's punishing you by locking

---

in many cases of thyroid disorders. I asked her to place one hand over that energy area while she tapped below that on the kidney meridian to clear away associated fears.

[55] This is a typical emotional release technique using AK/ Applied Kinesiology, where the point of pain or sensation is touched with one hand and the forehead Emotional Release Neurovascular points are covered with the other hand.

himself in there. You don't understand why he's in there. Breathe it all out."

At this point the emotional charge that Tanya felt was about a 5 on the scale of 0-10 around this memory. I asked what was the worst part of that memory for her that still had the most charge, and she responded that it was anger – a new emotion for her around this issue. She still felt some degree of sensation in her throat area.

I continued:

> "Hold one hand on your throat and go to the **Eyebrow Point**[56] to tap there. I want you to feel that little girl's confusion and frustration, and then a little bit of anger. Feel her frustration and confusion: 'Why did you do this? Why are you in there? Why did you leave me?' Then as an adult, imagine yourself saying: 'Come on out. It's okay. We're not going to hurt you. Come on out.' Just tap away that anger until you feel a shift. Breathe it out. Breathe out all the debris that you're clearing as you clear it. Breathe it out. It's okay to be angry. It's okay to let go of that anger. It's okay to feel angry that he had to go through what he went through to be as broken as he was, and then the rest of you had to suffer, too. Just breathe that out. He was doing the best he could do in every moment. That didn't make you feel any better or any more secure as a little girl. Breathe it out. Let it go. You deserved more love and more attention. You deserved to feel secure that your daddy wasn't going to leave you. He deserved to have more peace of mind instead of living his whole life with post traumatic stress. Just let go of it. It's all in the past. He's in a more peaceful place now and you can be, too. Just let it go. Breathe it out. You deserve to have peace of mind. Repeat: 'I choose to feel at peace.'"

I invited Tanya to go back to the two days that her dad locked himself in the room, and she reported that her emotional charge on that memory was down to zero and felt totally neutral.

---

[56] The EFT **Eyebrow Point** is located right above the nose where the hair of the eyebrow begins on both sides. You can use an index finger on one side and another finger on the other side while you lightly tap.

You will notice how in this work we focus on each separate aspect of an issue and tap away each emotion as it comes up using specific meridian tapping points. It usually does not take very long to bring the emotional charge down on an issue if it is the body's priority and the person is willing to go back and feel the emotion around the memory as she taps it away.

Based again on Tanya's written history, I guided her next to a younger age when she felt fearful that her dad was going to leave because he told her that he would. This was when her parents were not getting along, but then he couldn't get out of the driveway so he never did leave. After having tapped on the previous issue she had no charge left on this previously painful memory.

Thyroid Issues

At this point Tanya interjected that she wanted to switch the focus from her dad to her mom, saying that even though she'd actually worked on this memory before, she still had a charge of around 7 out of ten. The issue was that when her father had temper tantrums she felt a lot of emotional charge, and she said it seemed kind of comical in a way, because she remembers her mom would say nothing - absolutely nothing - which was probably good for the situation in the moment, but she stated that by her mother's example is how she learned to stuff her feelings and to say nothing. The image that came to her mind at this point was that she realized as a little girl she would stand there looking at her mother and wanting her mother to say something, wanting her to stand up to her dad and just tell him to stop the yelling. As a little girl she really wished that somebody had done something about it because she couldn't be the one. She felt helpless and very powerless, and that had followed her into adulthood in many areas of her life and health.

I proceeded to lead her as she continued **holding the throat/ thyroid area and forehead**.

> "Breathe that out. Just let go of that sense of having no power. Nobody listens to me. Mom isn't doing anything to change the situation. She won't tell him to stop. Just breathe that out."

I asked if she felt any anger toward her mother modeling for her to just stuff her feelings, and she responded yes, and that she held about a 6-7 charge on that anger toward her mom.

We continued:

> "Let's go there. How many years have you just not been able to say what you really feel? You couldn't when you were little. Your mom never said anything, for whatever reason, but she was a perfect model. You learned that your feelings didn't matter. Maybe doctors tell people with certain autoimmune symptoms: 'It's all in your head. It doesn't matter. It's not real. It's not showing up on the tests.' In this case, you had a lot of feelings. You didn't want your dad to yell anymore. You wanted him to behave. You didn't want to be walking on eggshells all the time. You wanted to be able to play and have fun and make noise if you wanted to, and you couldn't do that. You never knew when he was going to have a tantrum. You never knew when he was going to explode or what was going to make him explode. Your mom wouldn't do anything. She always held her emotions inside. You had to hold your emotions inside, too. Just breathe that out. All those years of bottled-up emotions, those can absolutely eat you up inside. Anybody with autoimmune knows that.
>
> Let's just breathe out all the stuff that we've all wanted to say in the past. I want everybody to hold your throat. This is your power center. This represents anything you've wanted to say in the past but you couldn't, anything you wanted to share, your feelings, your thoughts, your ideas, your dreams. Put the other hand across your forehead. All the things you wanted to share with your dad, Tanya, all the things you wanted to tell him, all the ways you wanted to be as a little girl but you couldn't because you didn't want to push his buttons and trigger him to go off. I'm sure even years later, you still couldn't tell your truth. You still couldn't share your emotions. You still had that stopper in there. You had learned so well to stuff how you felt, that your feelings didn't matter. It was all about dad."

Tanya added that the situation seemed to shift as she grew up, and her father got better, and he got happier and quit using. As an adult, what she realized was that she "just didn't even know who I was or even what I was feeling. I'm just detached from even knowing. It wasn't even a matter of stuffing emotions anymore. It's like I just didn't even know what I felt."

We continued the session with me facilitating:

> "Who is Tanya? What does Tanya feel? Are Tanya's feelings valid? Good questions. I'd like you to move your hand down to your **Third Chakra** or the solar plexus area, right around where your stomach and your small intestines and liver and gallbladder are, right in the middle below your breast. Leave the other hand across your forehead. I want you to breathe in the lost parts of yourself, the parts that went dormant, that got lost because you were focusing so much on the drama of your dad and your mom. Just breathe out that old story, the old habit, the old patterns of looking at life that way. Breathe that out. Breathe in all your lost parts and your own personal power. Breathe them in from all the old memories and all the places they've gotten lost. Breathe out all these other people that were more important than you and your feelings. Just breathe it out. One more breath, take a breath in. Feel it cleaning out all the old stuff that belonged to everybody else, putting everybody else's feelings and thoughts and needs first. Just breathe it all out.
>
> Next I want you to go to the points below your eyes, the **Under Eye Points**. Tap right there on the eye socket ridge. Tap right under your iris and pupil. I want you to think of all the stuff that you were carrying for your father and your mother, and maybe for your younger siblings from those days when Dad was still using and he was still having all this bottled-up anxiety and frustration. You were walking on eggshells and always putting him first, listening to his opinion, looking at how he acted instead of the way you acted, looking at how your mom reacted, and the fact that your feelings didn't seem to matter compared to their opinions and their feelings and their reactions. You were creating your own life and all of your reactions and all of your

behavior around them instead of what you wanted to do. Just breathe it out. It's their stuff and you can give it back. Just breathe out all those patterns, those stories, their reactions, and their needs and neediness. Let it all go. Just breathe it out.

Take a big breath in of your own energy and your own personal power. Feel it coming in and grounding you. Feel it filling up your body and going out through the bottoms of your feet into the earth so you can be grounded as yourself. Breathe out all this old stuff that belonged to your parents. Breathe in another big breath. Feel your own power coming back into you. Feel it going down your arms and out the tips of your finger. Feel it going all around in your trunk and down your legs, into your feet, down into the earth, and out the ends of your toes. Feel it shooting out the top of your head, completely filling you up with who you are as it expels all the stuff that belonged to everybody else that you put as more important than you. Breathe it all out. One more big breath in of pure personal power. Feel it glowing a bright white and gold. Feel it spinning inside of you as it breaks off all the old stuff from everybody else, all their shoulds and their patterns and their needs and their emotional outbursts and reactions and patterns. Blow it all out. Let it all go.

I want you to now move your fingers. Tap **Above and Below the Mouth**. You've got your index finger and middle finger horizontally tapping above and below your upper and lower lips. Tap those two points at the same time. Just focus on your own feelings and your own power now. How do you feel now looking back at your childhood? Any emotions or thoughts or comments come to mind?

Tanya replied, "It feels distant. I feel more present right now in my life, in this moment." She also mentioned that she no longer felt any anger toward her mother about learning from her to stuff emotions. She stated that she knew her mom was doing the best she could. She reported that the charge was gone around the anger but she still had a little sensation in her throat.

I mentioned that anytime she felt that "lump in the throat" or tightness in the throat she needed to go back to some of her "stuffed emotion" memories and to hold **one hand over her throat area and the other hand across her forehead** creating the Applied Kinesiology energetic circuit. With one hand on the neurovascular emotional release points and the other hand where the stuck emotion is located over the throat, the body can automatically clear the emotional blockage or charge.

Again using Tanya's history, I fast forwarded to her adult life and asked the following questions.

> "Do you have any anger right now about the birth of your first child or anything about that? You said you were angry because you couldn't hold him for two days, but it was a really traumatic birth process. Do you have any emotional charge about that now related to how you were treated in the hospital or how the baby was treated, or anything you would have really liked to tell the doctors?"

She responded that she had regrets about not being more assertive and felt angry at herself for not being more assertive. She said she felt a slight sensation or tightness in her chest area.

I focused now on clearing these emotional symptoms of dis-ease by asking Tanya to put **one hand on her chest** where she felt the sensation. I directed her to continue to tap **Above and Below the Mouth.** Sometimes we hold shame in these big meridians that go down the back and front. These tapping points can clear any embarrassment or shame associated with an issue or memory.

> "Tanya, maybe you were embarrassed to tell the doctor what you really felt. Maybe you were ashamed of anything about the birth process or your condition. Maybe you just felt guilty with the sadness of not being able to hold your child for a couple of days. Just breathe out all of those feelings. Because you weren't assertive, maybe you were more of a victim and so was your baby. That wasn't really your fault; it was the way you were conditioned. You're letting that go. That conditioning is gone and that will never be holding you back again.

Just breathe out all those old inner recordings of: 'You're not supposed to talk back to a doctor. You're not supposed to give an opinion. You're not supposed to tell them what you want. You're not supposed to be assertive.' Those people wear uniforms and you don't. They have initials after their name and you don't. Let go of all that. Breathe it out. They're humans just like you are. You deserve to be able to hold your baby. You deserve to be able to tell them how you felt. You have that birthright. It's time for you to be able to use that now. Breathe out all the inner blocks, the inner: 'I'm afraid to do it. I'm ashamed to do it. I'm embarrassed to do it. It might be dangerous for me to say something or be assertive. I might be abandoned or somebody may yell at me if I am assertive. Something bad might happen. I might get in trouble if I'm assertive.' Breathe that all out. Let it go.

Repeat after me:

I matter.

My opinions matter.

My emotions matter.

I choose to state what I need and what I want.

I choose to ask for behavior changes when necessary... like asking my dad to stop yelling."

At this point when I asked Tanya if she felt any more charge about being assertive she said she felt better about it and felt no charge. She added that she was even imagining herself holding her child in the NICU, breaking all the rules, and that felt good!

Tanya had originally stated in her history that she believed that her thyroid condition was her body's expression of the belief that she was not supposed to express who she was, what she thought, and what she felt. That lid on the personal power container was in her throat. She stated that it felt like a bottleneck that was too narrow and clogged. At this point she reported that the sensation in her throat had lowered to a 2 out of 10.

The **throat** is a power center or **chakra**. It is all about stating your truth, your opinion, your feelings; speaking your truth, or it can also represent not being allowed to state those things. Because the thyroid and parathyroid are located in the throat area, those are the glands that are going to be affected by stuck energy there. It makes perfect sense, right? In Tanya's case she felt like she hadn't mattered because her dad's needs always came first in her family, her opinions weren't listened to, her emotions were stuffed, and she really had no sense of self. This is a perfect example of how the body tries to send a message that it is time to state what needs to be said without keeping it bottled up anymore.

I suggested to Tanya that she continue to work on this area of her body that seemed to be her "weak link" where emotional stress could cause even more harm if it were not cleared. A natural way of letting the body clear stress from the throat area is to put one hand at the throat and one hand across the forehead. While doing this often the subconscious pushes forth unconscious thoughts, old memories, maybe dreams later. When they come to the surface they can be breathed out with the intention of clearing.

Tanya reported at this point that she felt more grounded than she had felt in over a month.

I recommended that she monitor any future sensations in her throat area and that we had covered enough for this session. As I closed the session I reminded her of the follow-up that ensured that she got the most from her session with me. I tell my clients the following to remember after every session when they use energy therapy to clear emotions:

> "After each session a good conscious thing to do is to consciously breathe out the old energetic ash that you have cleared. I highly advise that you take good care of yourself after an energy-clearing session like this. Drink lots and lots of water, at least for the next 24 hours during which time your meridians will recalibrate and shift per the energy work you have performed. Take an Epsom salt bath if you can. That helps with clearing the physical body memory and

allows the cells of the body and your largest organ, your skin, to clear. It's also cleansing for your auric field and your aura. It's very relaxing and helps with the recalibration of the electromagnetics of your biofield. So, for the next 24 hours, be gentle on yourself, get enough sleep tonight, and if you need to take a nap, feel free to do so. Don't overexert."

You may say that in this case I used just simple tapping, but anybody who's had a really deep, good, sobbing cry, knows how tired they are afterwards. That's the natural way the body lets go of emotional energy. What we did in this case is just as powerful and sometimes easier than having a good cry, but Tanya was still going to be tired as her body recalibrated. To end a session I talk more about space clearing and other techniques which are listed in my book focused on "best practices in energy management" that is available on my website or via Amazon.[57] I feel this is important because you don't want to walk right back into the energetic ash that you're burning off and letting go during an energy therapy session, so as a precaution it is advantageous to keep your space cleared.

---

[57] In my short Book, **EFT-Best Practices for Energy Management,** I also mention how you should talk to your electromagnetic biofield and subconscious mind, and how important it is to know how to work with both of these which we access via tapping on the meridians. Check out my book at: http://annemerkel.com/practitioner-publications/ or on Amazon at: http://is.gd/AnnesBooks

- Sally -

The subject most focused on during this case section is learning to **"Put yourself as number one"**.

When I work with autoimmune clients and people that have cancer and other serious issues, so often I see people that are wonderful caretakers, who are going out of their way, even during their illness, to take care of everybody else. I've had to literally sit down with some people with stage 4 cancer and have had to say: "Listen, I want to help you. It's time for you to focus on helping yourself. This is serious business here. It's your choice because I can't do the work for you. This is a matter of your life or death."

This is a regular talk I have with many people with serious autoimmune conditions that they've had for a long time. Once they decide that they want to live and get better, they realize they need to change some things about their lifestyle and their perception. Sometimes it's a matter of changing their belief system, too, as they look for more balanced ways to support themselves so that they can start to love themselves as number one. When they do this they can start to get better and later they can be more beneficial to all others in their lives.

If you've already been diagnosed, or even if you haven't but you know you've got autoimmune symptoms, you are on a road to degeneration unless you are taking good care of yourself first. There are many reasons why maybe that's a hard thing for you to do. You can be the detective and help yourself get well.

This is not easy for some people, and that's why I have so many clients who have autoimmune. They need support. They need help to make this shift. If you are a caregiver with family and friends and mates and children and parents and everybody that needs to be taken care of, remember that you really need to keep yourself as number one so that you can better serve these people, and you can stay well so that you can better support others.

Sally's Story

When I first started working with Sally she had left her job because she could no longer manage that with the physical conditions she suffered: **CFS/ Chronic Fatigue Syndrome** and **Fibromyalgia**.

Like so many others with these or similar autoimmune disorders, in her own words she reported the following symptoms which required that she make some dramatic life changes:

- "Brain fog
- Confused and easily overwhelmed
- Disorganized – can't remember where I've put things or what needs to be done (deadlines, etc.)
- Poor comprehension and lack of awareness – misunderstandings, mistakes, miss important information, miss telling people things they need to know
- Poor word-retrieval
- Slow: communication, response time, decision-making
- Difficulty getting up from seated position – very taxing
- Can't stand for more than two minutes and need to rest for long periods in-between: affects meal preparation, washing dishes
- Difficulty carrying small loads, e.g. laundry to washing machine
- Difficulty bending, leaning, getting down to the ground, e.g. changing sheets on bed, vacuuming, picking something up off the floor – very tiring/challenging
- Fatigue very easily
- Weakness: extending my arms, lifting small things. Using my arms for anything causes tiredness and fatigue, e.g. changing sheets, kitchen work, carrying groceries
- Suddenly tired and need to lie down/sleep
- At times feel like I'm going to pass out from tiredness
- Achey, sore muscles and painful joints – exacerbated by any activity
- After exercise, inert for two to three days and sore all over
- Easily overwhelmed, stress, panic, anxiety when I have to be somewhere at a certain time, travel, navigate, climb stairs in subway, triggered by all the noise, people, being underground, fluorescent lighting, social interactions.

- Very low productivity: able to perform 2-3 tasks a day, including cooking, dishes, cleaning, shopping, showering
- Dizziness
- Low energy – low functional compared to others – can't cope with schedules or having "to do"
- Virtually unable to manage day-to-day affairs: paperwork/phone calls, scheduling, finances, taxes, filing, mother's affairs, taxes, medical affairs, purchasing things I need. I can't remember where things are, conversations, where I've written things down
- It's a struggle to think ahead and plan – meals, navigating to a new doctor's office, difficulty anticipating what I'll need to know or bring
- Environmental sensitivities to city environment – want simplicity and quiet to feel calm and peaceful, to be in nature, quiet, fresh air
- Dry skin, dry hair, eczema, itchiness, reactions to mould, dampness, headaches, migraines, sore throats"

We worked together to clear the emotional causes of her physical and mental symptoms. Some of the emotions she reported initially that she was fighting inside of herself included:

> "... lots of fear, stress, resistance, shame, humiliation, grief come up over the past year around making mistakes, being a mistake, and/or being mistaken, believing I am responsible for fixing all mistakes by myself, being deeply flawed and fearful that others will not like me when they discover this, thinking the illness is my fault, self-blame and self-criticism (why can't I just get on with it and get a job?), fear of putting myself out there, exposing my stuff, failing, losing everything, not being able to create a life for myself, being unwanted, not having financial independence, fear around boundaries being violated, not being able to stand up for myself, needing permission and approval from others, fear of men, being alone, abandoned, being impossible to live with because I'm a bad person or pathetic, rejection of being a woman, fear of being betrayed, not having a right to be alive, living a dying, being disabled, helpless and helpless."

Do these feelings sound familiar? I've seen these emotions show up many times in cases like Sally's, and my protocol is usually to focus on clearing the charge around the local or present physical or psychological symptoms and then clear the basic causes.

Sally was diligent in her work to clear the issues and she was soon feeling much better and able to get out more and start to create a new life for herself.

Sally's Next Challenge

At this stage of Sally's case she and I focused on a new aspect of her life as she began a one-on-one relationship with another person suffering from physical issues. I invited Sally to briefly provide an overview of what was going on:

> "I'm 53 and I've had autoimmune since I was 18. I managed it most of my life on my own and managed to work fulltime. Just last spring I really crashed. I just couldn't function anymore. My symptoms had been getting steadily worse with stress and stuff. I've been off work since last year, no income. I've been determined to spend the time looking at my own emotional issues and my mental beliefs and thought patterns. I already had a good diet, but I've been improving my diet and seeing a naturopath. Basically over the past year I was spending a lot of time focusing on watching inspiring videos and doing activities that really helped to bring me to a place of peace and balance out my emotions. That was taking up a very large chunk of my time. It was working and I was very happy and felt really good a lot of the time. Just in the last few months I went through a lot of change.
>
> About two and a half months ago I started a new relationship. That amped everything up to a whole other level. What I now come to see is that I have to relearn the practice of self-care in the context of relationship. I've been overtaxing myself trying to spend time with this person and adjusting to a relationship in general. Also it's been triggering really big, unconscious behaviors in me which are geared to taking care of other people first. I guess I just reached a crisis with that and I've been extremely depressed the last few days, just trying to understand why it's so

important to me that I get some kind of sense of worthiness out of relieving other people's pain and suffering. What I realize is that what I actually need to do is use relationship as a mirror to see that it's my own pain and suffering that I need to keep working on. Like Anne says, it's an ongoing thing for the rest of my life that I have to put into daily practice."

Sally had done a good job clearing many layers of both DNA-inherited emotional trauma as well as first hand life trauma, and her initial symptoms had abated to a large extent. She wisely saw this new relationship as a challenge and a trigger, and she was ready to move one and through her old emotional patterns as classic care-taker.

I invite you to think about the relationships that you are currently in. How much of yourself do you give to other people? How often does that really tax your system? You might say or think things such as: "I have to do this for others," or "I had to end up getting out of a marriage to support my health," or "I had to give up a lifestyle and a work situation and change my career because of the condition." Each story is unique, however there are some universal patterns that can help us all when we become aware of them.

In Sally's case this new relationship with her boyfriend reflected back a history of how she had taken care many other significant people in her life including her dad and boss. She also shared that sometimes the issues that her boyfriend triggered reminded her of issues that her mom and ex-husband had exhibited.

Sally reflected to me:

"I learned to take care of my mother from a very young age. It's conditioned into me. It's like a reaction that I have where I just step in with people I'm in primary relationships with. I don't do it with friends so much, although we can do it in a mutual exchange kind of supportive way. I sort of had this cycle with my mother trying to relieve her suffering but only receiving resentment from her that I was trying to help her. That's been a big pattern that I've been working on and looking at."

Meridian Tapping Away Relationship Stress Related to Caretaking Wounds

If you can relate to Sally's pattern of taking care of everyone else – even without appreciation or focus on her own needs, then I invite you to tap along at the **Heart Center** with the index finger on the Thymus Point and the other three fingers of one hand in a vertical line between your breasts. Because you're tapping along your central meridian over your heart chakra, and you're including the thymus, which is all about the immune system, this is really good for accessing and clearing deep emotional or belief patterns.

Think back to your early life and the people that you took care of or you felt like you had to protect. Continue tapping as you scan your memory bank for any emotional charge associated with your care-taking at an early age and beyond.

I asked Sally to think about how she tried to protect her mom from her dad. In my case, my mother manifested serious back problems as the way she dealt with her emotional issues growing up, so we always had to take care of mommy. I'm sure many people can really relate to this. A lot of us had others in our lives who just shut down or who had addictions that allowed them to "exit" from life and maybe from you. Think of ex-spouses or other people in your life that you have had to support when they exited through drugs or alcohol or depression, or they just didn't show up emotional or didn't come home physically.

Tap out the stress of living with or being around these people and feeling somewhat responsible for taking care of their weaknesses. As you tap just feel your own stress, frustration, sadness, sense of abandonment, or other emotions, and breathe them all out. Let go of the old emotional blocks that continue to hold you down and keep you sick.

As you tap, focus on the pain you felt growing up, that these people:
- were not there, or
- you couldn't help them, or
- you couldn't reach them, or
- they were not there for you, or

- even when you tried to protect them and save them they didn't notice or appreciate your diligence and caring.

If it's difficult to tap on the **Heart Center**, tap on the **Karate Chop** *Point* on the side of your hand.

Here I continue to guide your thought process based on Sally's case... as you continue tapping away any old emotional debris.

> "As you tap, realize that you were offering good service. You were offering good heart energy through your action. You were reaching out to really support and help somebody. They were unable to receive your blessings. They were unable to receive just the blessing of you being there with them and caring about them. They were so broken that they just couldn't thank you. They just couldn't acknowledge what a great job you were doing. If you were young, you didn't know that. You couldn't figure that out. You just knew that you were trying your best and nobody appreciated it. In fact, you sometimes got in trouble for it.

> Focus on how that feels. If you have a sensation in your body where you actually feel this energy stuck physically, then put one hand over that location and the other hand across your forehead, above your eyebrows where the emotional release points are. Just feel that feeling and breathe it away until it either moves, and then you follow it with that one hand, or it goes away. Breathe out all those times you have done your best, all those times you have offered help and support to somebody else, and all the times you haven't been accepted, you haven't been thanked, you haven't been acknowledged for doing that. Just tap it out and breathe it away.

> Next I want you to go to the fact that maybe you even hurt yourself in trying to help somebody else. You got in trouble. Maybe you were punished. Maybe you overexerted as you were trying to help somebody else. Maybe you had a lot of sleepless nights or you had a lot of worry, or you got into a situation with the wrong people because you were trying to help somebody else. You put yourself in jeopardy of their

anger or somebody else's abuse, or you just forgot to take care of yourself at that point, early in your life, when you tried so hard to take care of somebody else. You started this pattern of not getting supported for the good work you were doing, and feeling very worthless, feeling like your purpose was to help and nobody was appreciating it, nobody was open, nobody was receiving your gifts. It was a like a slap in the face. Just focus on that aspect if any of it pertains to your case.

Maybe people don't believe in how you're helping them. Maybe they don't want to be helped. They're so depressed that they just can't get out of depression. Or maybe they feel like they deserve to be punished. Maybe their religious convictions or their own worthiness issues and upbringing tell them that they deserve to suffer. They deserve to be in a situation without love. When you send them love, they can't receive it or they push it away; they may rebuke you for trying to send them something that they don't know how to receive or that they feel is wrong for them to receive. This can be very hurtful to you. Think about any cases where that relates to you and just tap those away. Breathe out all that hurt, disappointment, frustration. Just breathe it out.

Often times this old hurt comes up when you visit a person or a family member from your past during a family reunion or a holiday, where all the old memories with corresponding emotional charge comes boiling up. You may then find yourself still trying to help these people and they're still pushing you away. They may even be laughing at you. They're telling you your ideas are wrong, or they're not going to accept them, saying: "Don't waste my time. Mind your own business." You're still just trying to help. Breathe out these retorts and the inner hurt that you feel, and just let go of the charge. These people don't know any better... and they probably will never learn to appreciate the gifts you are offering them by just being you and trying to help and serve. You offer what you know could help them, but their fear and resistance won't let you help. Maybe on some level they're feeling that they don't deserve help. They seem to be pushing you away, but it's not really them: it's the situation, their belief system, and what they learned growing up. Just let the old stories and memories go. Breathe them out and resolve to someday go back and use your imagination to create happy endings to those memories, where these people finally do wake up and realize what a big help you are, how much you've saved them grief, and how much energy you give to them. In the meantime, move on with your life!"

I hope you are still tapping on your meridian points: either the **Heart Center** or **Karate Chop**. Back to Sally...

"Now I want you to think about all the people in your life that you have gotten close to. As you got closer to them you realized they needed help or support. By going into their private life, information, private thoughts, problems, with an open heart, sometimes you got hooked into their feelings. It's like the saying "you can lead a horse to water but you can't make them drink." We've all led our personal friends, family members, loved ones to water. Often they've refused to drink. Sometimes it's safer for your health and wellbeing to not get too involved before it's too late, or to get out before you begin to physically suffer or die.

I knew a woman who had already battled cancer. She knew that her boyfriend, her lover was bad for her health. She always had flare-ups when she was around him. He pushed her buttons and he upset her. I had a talk with her and said: "This is killing you." She said: "I know. Being with him is killing me, but I'm really having a hard time staying away." She later died because she couldn't disconnect. It takes a lot of courage to truthfully see what around you is bad for you and to pull away from that."

Sally had done a good job of protecting herself in the past. She had pulled away from a husband and a working situation that really were killing her. Now she had to decide about this new relationship that was pushing her life out of balance and bringing back physical symptoms.

Can you remember a case in your life where it was difficult to pull away from a person or situation, or where even though it was difficult you did it? Maybe you're still in a situation that you know is unhealthy for you. Maybe this is an unhealthy diet or an unhealthy work setting. Maybe it's an unhealthy relationship with somebody. Whatever it is, only you can solve your problem, and that involves changing the circumstances, your perception, or environment within the situation.

Sally made an astute observation at this point in her session:

> "I see clearly now how maybe this is something that people with autoimmune might all have in common. My own vulnerability, insecurity, and weakness is something that I have always tried to push away and have rejected in myself, and I felt very ashamed of this. That shame has prevented me from really being there for myself and giving myself compassion and acceptance when I needed it. Realizing that today, I see my relationships in a very different perspective. That insecurity was coming up strongly at those times when my boyfriend wasn't able to be available for me. I was taking his absence very personally when in fact it was just because he was having his own disconnect with his own problems with autoimmune or trauma or whatever. I don't need to fix him, I just need to continue to have my own self-care routine and just to give myself the time to be with all of these vulnerable emotions that do come up. When you grow up in families where your vulnerability becomes a liability, you try to hide it and disconnect from it. It just seems like that's an important piece of this for me to understand."

I think a golden rule that we all need to remember, that Sally pointed out, is that "if you feel it, it's in you." Nobody else is making you feel a certain way. They may be triggering, but they're triggering a button that's already in you. You are being guided to learn energy clearing tools to clear that button so that soon they can keep doing whatever they want and it won't bother you. It's their stuff. As long as you have a weakness or an emotional button, and you feel something or are triggered, then not only is it in you, but you are vulnerable to anybody else until you clear it.[58]

---

[58] For more information about this concept, go to: Ryce, Michael, ND. (1997) **Why is This Happening to Me... Again?!... and What You Can Do About It!** Theodosia, Missouri: dr. michael ryce, whyagain@kcmo.com .

We all need to remember that everybody is doing the best that he or she can do in every moment... even if that is not too good. I think once we really get that, then we can all more easily forgive. We're all human. None of us are walking on air yet. We're still living in human bodies, which indicates that we still have emotional baggage to clear.

As a child Sally tried to help her mom who basically said: "Forget it. You're putting me up on a pedestal and I don't belong there. Don't waste your effort." As a child she took that as a horrible slap in the face that really, really hurt. I'm sure that you can think of somebody that you really care about or some experience where people just have not accepted who you are or what you offer and how hurtful that's been.

In her present new relationship she was fighting a lot of depression and the feeling of her boyfriend pulling away and going into his own stuff. Her old neglect, desertion, and really wanting to help issues were coming up, but he didn't recognize how much she was giving him in the relationship, so was still pushing her away.

After all of this tapping I asked Sally how she felt at this point, and she responded:

> "Much, much better. The work you did with me has been a huge help. I guess I'm really lucky because I'm experiencing some very new things in this relationship that I haven't had before. My boyfriend is actually a very loving and caring person when he's not in his space of shock or trauma, which does come up for him, as it does for all of us at times. He didn't experience any compassion in his family at all, so he needs to do some work to develop compassion for himself. I guess I just can step back now and see that that's just where he's at. He told me a story about an extremely traumatizing event and went into shock. Then the next day, he just went into denial about it. I found that very distressing, but I just realized that that was where he needed to be at that time. It had nothing to do with me. Although it can be frustrating and it's okay for me to express that, I feel that it was much more about my own needs and insecurities about feeling

abandoned by him. I felt I just took on all this stuff. I personalized a lot. I'm not personalizing at all now. He's not perfect by any means, and he does need to get some help. I'm certainly not perfect either. He's there and he's not abandoning me at all. He has his moments where he's not connected, but he's not intentionally abandoning me in any way. He's really there to the best of his ability. That's the main thing for me."

I acknowledged Sally by saying:

"You are walking in uncharted waters. You were in a marriage and you got out of that. You left a difficult job where you were expected to "take care of" the boss. You've been taking good care of yourself lately. You have been diligent about trying to get well and choosing that you're going to spend time working on your issues and your health. Now you have the courage to get into a relationship and notice what a mirroring situation that is, as are all relationships... where once people get close to you start pushing your buttons."

That's a requirement of a relationship - to provide a catalyst for evolution. That's where even the best of relationships require some support of ourselves and some backing up and clearing another issue, another layer. It is an ongoing thing, and is a blessing that relationships can bring to all of us, too. Everybody around us is human. We all have issues. We can help each other to get beyond and clear our own stuff. Sally and others like her are definitely doing a courageous thing.

I said this to Sally at the end of our session and I want to share with you that when you feel like you're taking a step and you need more courage such as in backing away from caretaking or starting to focus on yourself as number one, the **Collarbone Point** or meridian K27 kidney point[59], is a good place to tap away your fear. Whenever you think that an action may require more courage on your part, tap there. Whenever you need to step into a new place, just tap there and breathe in courage while you breathe out fear.

---

[59] These points are at the base of your throat on both sides, below the collarbones, at the beginnings of the first ribs.

Fear can really stop you in your tracks, keep you sick, and keep you stressed. You don't need fear, so tap it away!

Another thing I want to share here is that when you are sensitive and when you're helping other people as caregivers, you may take on energy and hurt from those people. The typical place where we store that is the stomach meridian. The tapping point for that is **Under the Eye**. It's right on the edge of the eye socket rim, under the eye, right below the iris and the pupil. Take one hand and with your thumb and one finger, you can tap on both **Under Eye** points. As you're doing that, think of the people you've been with and clear any energy you have picked up from them.

I have seen so many cases of cancer patients who spent a lot of time around other people with cancer prior to getting sick. They basically took on the energy of cancer and they attracted it into their bodies. Every day you need to clear your energy field and clear stuff that you've taken on from others. It's very nice to be sympathetic and be there for your friends that are having problems in their lives, but remember that it helps nobody for you to carry their problems or worries to the extent that you take on their pain.

If you are an empathetic person, it's not helping the other person for you to take on their stuff. It surely doesn't help you to carry their burden. Many of us have carried our parents' burdens for our whole life. Every feeling our mother had while she was pregnant with us, everything that anybody felt around us until we were about age ten, we have just soaked it up. We carry it until we consciously clear it. Tap **under the eyes** and consciously say: "I choose to clear this hurt that my mother had, this anger my mother had, anger my father had, this insecurity, depression, disease, sad story, etc." Give yourself permission to let go of the stuff that you take on that doesn't belong to you. There's really no need to suffer.

So, I hope that Sally's case is a good reminder of life attitudes and skills that can help you to become more powerfully balanced and to stay healthy... even as you take care of others in your life.

- Amanda -

We as humans are continuing to learn about this beautiful physical body that we're in, and learn why it's hurting itself from the inside out. In this section let us look at some of the causes of why the physical symptoms have come out: specifically the emotional causes as we worked with **Amanda.**

As I relate Amanda's case, I'd like you to remember that anytime you're working with your meridians, it is beneficial. You might not see the direct, exact, immediate results that you have as your priority, but you're always supporting your body in its priorities. I tell this to all of my clients, because often the results are very subtle, or some issues will clear quickly and easily while others may take longer or must be cleared in segments as we focus on one aspect of the issue at a time... when the body deems that you are ready to clear it. Your body's priorities always take a higher position than anything you want the body to do.

Amanda's Case

When Amanda presented to me first during a live **Autoimmune Coaching & Energy Therapy Support** call,[60] and I asked her to start tapping at the **Heart Center** points while she shared her history. She introduced herself and her situation by saying the following:

> "I have **Wegener's Vasculitis.** It started about three years ago, so a year prior to my diagnosis I was chronically tired, chronic infections. I was getting blood blisters, tonsil infections, ear infections. Long story short, summer of 2012 I was sick to the point that my kidneys were failing, my liver enzymes were up, my lungs were -- they believed I had pneumonia. I was admitted to the hospital with pneumonia and that's when my lungs collapsed. They put me in an induced coma for 14 days. That's where they diagnosed that I have Wegener's Vasculitis, which is where the blood flow

---

[60] Learn more about this series at:
http://www.myeftcoach.com/autoimmune-coaching-support-group/

gets cut off to major organs. The vessels almost swell to the point that they burst. It can be fatal.

From there, luckily, by the grace of God, I survived 28 days in the hospital. Treatment was high, high doses of prednisone and cyclophosphamide, which is chemo. The thing with the disease is you never really know what causes it -- they argue that it's either something genetic or a viral or bacterial infection. The fact that I was really sick kind of leading up to it, leading a very busy, stressful life, not really sure what played into that. The symptoms when I was in …. It's a little painful to talk about.

As soon as I got out of the hospital I had six months of chemo treatments, a year of prednisone. I just finished a year of methotrexate. Now I'm going to be starting another drug just for maintenance purposes. I have been fortunate to be in remission for about a year. The thing with the disease is you never know when it's going to flare, when it's going to come back. They watch all the things closely. My current symptoms, there's a thing called ANCA that they watch to see, if that number increases, it's a possibility that my body is starting to flare up. For the last couple months, for some reason, that number is coming back up. All my typical blood work seems to be stable, so I'm not really sure why that's happening. I've noticed that I do have increased tiredness. I have seen a few small blood lesions kind of come up. I do have a little bit of eczema. I retain tons of water. I'm still dealing with the side effects from the medication. If I was in an acute flare, my lungs could start bleeding, my kidneys could start failing, blood blisters, and basically any major organ can become compromised."

At this point I'd like to share a bit about Amanda's history as she provided it to me in her pre-coaching form.

Amanda was under super stress. She had a job and was getting ready for a new job, which she started right before getting very sick. She was in school taking courses and she had been taking them ever since to finish her degree. Amanda had smoked for 14 years even though as a child she'd had asthma. She had been giving up smoking because she had a two-year-old. She acted as guardian of her handicapped brother even though he was being taken care of in a facility at that time. Six months prior to all the symptoms, Amanda had had a miscarriage. She and her husband were trying to have another child. At that time, she had related that her diet was full of dairy, gluten, anything she felt like eating.

She was leading quite a busy and stress-filled life: in school, working, tending a two-year-old, trying to get pregnant leading to a miscarriage, and then giving up smoking on top of all of that. All of these things were not only stressful physically but also mentally, emotionally, and spiritually, too. She remarked that many people were not surprised when she became ill.

But, Amanda was used to a life full of stress. She told me in her history that she had always been kind of a perfectionist. At a young age, she pretty much had to take care of her mother and brother, who had some handicaps. It seems she never really had a childhood.

Generally one has to change one's life in order to survive serious autoimmune issues. This requires creating a new lifestyle with new attitudes. A rebalancing must occur as you're planning ahead and thinking ahead. For Amanda, as well as a lot of others, her symptoms in the past had been so serious that survival was the biggest issue.

Yet, Amanda had a to-do list that was very intense. She said that her goals were:
- to finish her degree very soon after our first session,
- to get back to work directly after that, and
- to have another baby... when her present child was almost five years old at the time.

Just a couple of years after her major illness event she had a family, a child, was guardian to her handicapped brother, was still studying, anticipating her next job, and then still planning to get pregnant. This girl was driven,... but was that in her best interests?

Amanda provided more information about her situation:

"The job that I actually quit before I really got sick wasn't a good environment. It was very stressful. It wasn't the work that was stressful; it was the people. In fact, the reason why it got so bad is because I was sick all the time. Sadly, I lost credibility and people thought I wasn't reliable. Who would have thought that my body was starting to fall apart, right? I am looking to return to human resources which was what my degree is in.

I decided to be very picky in terms of that. I think the breaking point, too, was the work and school. That is why I have not returned to work until this school is done, because I knew that that was a key. I can't do that. I have very much the expectation that in a perfect world I'll find something four days a week. Outside of my son, that's about all I will be doing."

Amanda's case is like so many others. The symptoms start to come on but there may not be an indication that it is very serious until too late.

I continued to delve into her case for more clues as to when the stresses of life started to take their toll, and it starts to show up pre-birth.

Potentially there was a lot of trauma carried in Amanda's DNA because her mother had suffered a lot of abuse and trauma in her childhood. Because she didn't really have a decent family life growing up, she seemed to want to create a family to make her happy. There were a lot of expectations on Amanda, who related that her birth was normal but that she didn't start breathing for a few minutes after she was born. She admitted that maybe there was a bit of subconscious reluctance to arriving into the situation in which she was born.

Amanda's parents divorced when she was five. Her mother started seeing other men even though she got married again. Amanda knew that there was some cheating going on behind her step father's back. Then there was a second divorce when she was nine. Her mother was into all kinds of shenanigans and cheating and lying so she did not really have a relationship with her at the time of her illness, and had said goodbye to that relationship.

Amanda did comment that around the time of our session her mother had requested that they go to a counselor together, saying that she was persistent and promised she would change. Amanda noted that she was skeptical, and also noticed that after that request was when she started to see symptoms return.

We all have parents and they are humans who have stuff that they've inherited from their parents, who have inherited from their parents, and so it goes. We get lots of emotional and psychological input from the DNA of our ancestors. Our parents do the best they can do, just like we do the best we can do in every moment. But, some parents have been really horrible, so there is a lot of stuff to clear, even though they may have had intentions of trying to be good parents.

Working with Amanda – Her First Session

When I asked Amanda to focus on when she was a little girl and her mother was doing things that she knew were not right, while expecting her to take care of her and her brother - to be responsible for their health and well-being, Amanda said she felt pressure in her chest.

I asked her to put one hand right where she felt it in her chest with the other hand across her forehead in a kinesiological hold while she thought of the issues during childhood related to her mother. She said that she felt guilty a lot and felt her mother's anger. Her mom was abusive sometimes. She screamed and got really angry, yelling at her stepfathers and probably her father when she was very young. She had had a really hard childhood, but she was bringing a lot of her angst into Amanda's childhood. This brought up lots of sadness in Amanda and she began to cry.

I guided her through some tapping to clear the sadness that arose and her sense of loss of her childhood. After she reported that she felt relieved of that, we continued.

At that point I took her to another point that she had brought up in her history involving a car accident at age 15 when she was driving.

Even though nobody was hurt in the accident, she reported that she still felt a high level of guilt about the incident. She stated that she felt a 10 on a scale of 0 to 10... even after many years.

I asked Amanda to tap the points **Above and Below the Mouth** first while she focused on that guilt. I asked whether there was something she would like to say to those in the car during the accident , to get it off her chest and let go of some of the guilt. She replied:

> "I'd like to say that I'm sorry. I did say sorry during all of that. The biggest issue is that we were all underage -- I didn't have a driver's license. The older friends of ours, kind of covered it up, so it was a big lie. They said I wasn't driving.
>
> They were good friends – and they still are. I'm still friends with them, but I still feel terrible about it."

We did some meridian tapping on:

> "I choose to let go of this guilt. It's unbeneficial for everybody else.
>
> I choose to let go of this guilt.
>
> I choose to accept that it was a stupid thing that I did when I was 15.
>
> I choose to understand that everybody riding with me made a silly mistake, too.
>
> I understand that guilt is a heavy emotion that can really keep me stuck."

Amanda continued tapping until she felt a shift and a lifting of the guilt.

Guilt can be something that really can make a big impact. It can impact your self-esteem, your sense of self-worth. It can really keep a person paralyzed. In Amanda's history, that was a significant trauma that she had listed, and I wanted to see if we could clear that before going on. At this point she reported that she felt the guilt had lowered in intensity to about a 3 from a 10.

She reported that she still felt it a bit in her stomach, which was normal for her whenever she thought of the accident. I asked Amanda to place her hand where she felt it in her stomach and the other hand across her forehead in a kinesiological hold. She did this and then looked back over the memory of the event. She then reported that she felt no more guilt about the accident.

So, we went back to her mom issues and I asked about what she felt then when she thought about her mom. She reported a fear of being lied to again, and again she felt the sensation in her chest. She created the energetic circuit using the kinesiological hold with her hands across her forehead and on her chest. I asked that she go back to the negative emotions she felt about her mom during the most traumatic memory she could think of, with the worst repercussions related to her mom's lies. She chose a memory with a charge of 10 out of 10 on the 0 to 10 scale related to abandonment.

Amanda's mother had been abandoned and Amanda had inherited the predisposition to feel abandoned, plus, her mother had abandoned her when she went off on her tangents and when she told lies about where she was going, where she had been, or when she might return.

I invited Amanda to tap on her **Karate Chop Point** on the side of her hand or at her **Heart Center**. She tapped on:

> "You're feeling all alone.
>
> You can't even trust your mother.
>
> Who can you trust if you can't trust your mother?
>
> That hurt you so much.
>
> Why couldn't she tell you the truth?
>
> You felt so alone and so responsible for other people.

Who was taking care of Amanda?"

Amanda felt the energy shift and reported the charge had come down from a 10 to a 4, and now she felt angry about the abandonment.

At this point I asked Amanda to place one hand over her chest where she had it before and with the other hand, I asked her to tap at the end of her eyes, on the gallbladder **End of Eye** EFT point, or I like to explain that this is where Cleopatra draws her long eyeliner toward the temple. I asked her to go in there to that memory and feel the anger.

"I was abandoned.

I was lied to.

Where were you when I needed you?

I was always there for you, but where were you when I needed you?

You were supposed to be the mother.

That really hurts.

That really makes me angry.

I feel angry about it.

Mom, I'm so angry that you did that back then.

I've been carrying that for so many years.

That hurt.

I choose to let it go.

It's nasty energy that I've been carrying."

Amanda reported that the emotional charge on that nasty memory was down to a zero. I asked her to go to another traumatic memory where she was lied to by her mother. She summarized:

> "My mother continued this into my adult life, so shortly after I woke up from the coma, I could tell that she was seeing another boyfriend while married."

She said that she felt disgusted that her mother always seemed to have a guy on the side, and that she felt it in her gut.

While tapping **Above and Below the Mouth**, right above her upper lip and below her lower lip, she felt the shame that she had felt for her mother since she was a little girl, with that sense of disgust, shame, and embarrassment. After tapping she said she felt better.

I asked her to go back to that time when she was waking up from the coma and there was her mom who she knew was lying then. On a scale of 0 to 10 she reported that she only now felt a 1 or 2 about that.

When I asked Amanda to think back in general about her mom wanting to get back in contact, wanting to be in her life, she said the worst feeling before was the fear of being lied to and that was a 10, but now it was a 3 or 4.

I told Amanda that her mom might still lie to her, but her charge was different so it wouldn't affect her as much. The important thing was that she wouldn't be walking around with that high-level charge that might cause undue stress in Amanda every time her mother mis-behaved or lied.

Many people have others in their lives, and they just can't carry any more of the "emotional baggage" for these people. In fact, they've got a lot of stuff in their aura and in their energy field that doesn't belong to them, and that can lead to ill health. Tapping the **Under the Eye Points** is very therapeutic on a regular basis just to clear other people's stuff. There are a lot of energy-suckers out there, and I advised Amanda to make a habit of clearing her mother's stuff out of her own system. We started by tapping on the following:

"It's unbeneficial for me to still be carrying my mother's emotions.

This stuff really hurts me.

It never benefitted my mother either.

It's time to clear this energy.

I choose to let go of her energy now.

I choose to cut the cords to my mother.

I send them back with love and gratitude to where they came from.

I choose to be cleared totally of my mother's influence and her emotions.

I choose to be cleared totally of my mother's emotions and baggage and influence.

I choose to reclaim my personal power.

I choose to let go of my mother's influence.

I choose to let go of my mother's pain.

I choose to let go of my mother's trauma and abandonment issues.

I choose to allow my body to heal itself."

On a scale of 0 to 10 Amanda reported the charge was down to a 0 or 1 and that she felt much lighter. She added that she felt a bit drained, but not too bad. She also said that the thought of her mother coming back into her life no longer caused her to feel panic inside. The charge was down to around a 1 out of 10.

Amanda wanted to know if what we did was permanent or if the emotional charge would return. I responded:

"What we did and the aspects we cleared are clear, but other aspects may come up. The analogy that I like to use is that of the beautiful gemstone, a diamond with the facets. Each facet or gemstone surface represents an aspect of the issue at hand. The work we do clears a few aspects at a time. There may still be a few facets or surfaces that we haven't seen on the diamond. They're not pointed in the direction we've been working in, so we can't see them yet. They may show up at some point, and then you can clear them alone or with a facilitator. These additional aspects of the original issue will probably hold less emotional charge because you've taken the edge off of the whole issue. The basic stuff we've worked on and the way we've worked on it should be gone."

Then Amanda asked if I thought her physical symptoms would abate based on our work in this short session, to which I replied:

"That's a real good question for your situation, and it's really up to the body. Where was that guilt about your car accident working in your system in relation to all your symptoms? We don't know. Only the body knows. Where was that panic and fear of your mother and fear of being lied to again? Where was that playing a part?

We didn't even work on your physical symptoms. We didn't work on your skin issues. There are some big issues that if we would work together one on one, I'd want to go in and clear. For example, your lung meridian and your large intestine meridian would both be a real high priority, and your kidney and bladder meridians. We really didn't go into any of those today.

What I wanted to do is go to some of the specifics that you mentioned because you did mention them. They are all part of the whole person that you are, Amanda. In answer to your question, you may feel some shifts in your symptoms. You may feel a lightness. You may notice that some aspect of your life just gets easier. You are on another drug, so you're not quite sure what the reaction of your body on that drug is. I will say that anybody doing energy therapy like we're doing right now who is using medication will get more of the positive benefits from those medications. They'll do what they're supposed to be doing more than if you've got a lot of blockage. A chiropractic adjustment will hold better if you're clearing the emotional stuff first. Herbs and natural remedies and homeopathy will work better. Any kind of treatment that you're getting will be supported by us clearing this energy that is deep inside of you and in your subconscious and your electromagnetic biofield."

Amanda's Follow-up Session

Amanda and I ended up working together for one month – a total of four sessions after the first one. Then after four months I worked with her again on another **Autoimmune Coaching & Energy Therapy Support** call.

Amanda again introduced herself:

> "Two and a half years ago I was diagnosed with an autoimmune disease called Wegener's Vasculitis. It's an attack of the small blood vessels that can swell up and cut off blood supply to my organs. Long story short, it landed me with pneumonia in the hospital, and that put me in a coma for 14 days in a total of a 28-day hospital stay. From that I was given chemo and massive steroids. That kind of led me to looking at additional options to help heal myself.
>
> I had a lot of trauma from being put in a coma for 28 days. And, I had just had a miscarriage. My last job was stressful because I missed so much work because my body was shutting down. I didn't feel good about myself and my productivity in that job. That left some bad feelings. I was also a student at the time working on a degree. I was doing all kinds of things, working, working on the degree, trying to get pregnant, and then my body just said: 'Enough! Uncle! I'm not putting up with this.' And I also had a young three-year-old child at the time."

That is an awful lot for any person to take on all at one time. I asked Amanda what had changed in her life during the short time we had worked together. She responded:

> "Lots of things have shifted. The disease is completely in remission, so that's great. Through the EFT I've cleared lots of trauma around the disease and the fear about it. Even trigger words such as 'since I had chemo,' and that kind of stuff, would really send me off. And also around past, growing up, in my childhood, issues with my mother, lots of stuff has shifted. I've been able to let go and just kind of move on from lots of issues. On top of that, I started looking at other things like diet and exercise and what else I could do. You mentioned, of course, the Paleo diet, which has been very, very helpful. Since I started two months ago – forgive me, I've had blurps because of vacation and Christmas, but I've lost over 17 pounds of the 75 that I gained taking steroids. That's been huge for me. And I know that it works. I know going forward that's got to be a main component in my life.
>
> After Christmas and everything that had transpired, I had finished my degree. I did get very tired. I can correlate my tiredness directly to the Paleo diet, which I had somewhat dropped over the Holiday.
>
> When I did that those symptoms kind of came back, but I think the difference in me then and me before was I could recognize what was causing the symptoms. It was like: 'Okay, calm down. You know the diet worked before so it's time to get back on it.' And then different things kind of came into play. That includes the eating better and the sleeping and just going back to simple things that made me feel better, including tapping, of course."

I asked Amanda what were her goals for this follow-up session and she replied:

> "I want to focus on the future. I think that once I can get back to work, I'm back finally. I think I have some fear around that. I think I have fear about being able to juggle working again and family. I know deep down I'm more than ready. I think it's just my own feelings of how things went

down when I got sick that's holding me back."

Often when the physical symptoms go away, the thought of getting on with life can be full of doubts such as: "Is it going to come back? Am I up to this? What am I going to do?"

I know a lot of people have fear of moving forward with their life that basically keeps them sick. They're afraid to get well because then they will have to face potentially going back to a bad or stressful job, an industry that they don't like anymore, or a lifestyle that didn't work for them before, but they think they have to go back to it now. There are a lot of different ways that people keep themselves in the suffering mode. Amanda didn't do that – she got herself well. Luckily she had support from her husband to at least pay the bills as she was healing. Now it was time to move forward and find a job without blocking herself from that. The last job didn't give a great recommendation for Amanda because she was falling apart. That happens a lot with people developing autoimmune disorders.

With those of us who suffer from autoimmune disorders, we live not with a "life sentence of suffering", but with a "life sentence of living a different kind of life than the typical society lives". We can't eat the foods that they eat because that will make us sick. We might not be able to work in the same kind of job as we used to because it might have been so stressful that that's what made us sick. We've got to change the kind of relationships we've been in if they have been stressful or energy-draining. The work that I do with clients helps them get beyond this so that changing life patterns isn't as painful as it might have been. And, the beauty of using energy therapy and natural health tools is that individuals learn to use these on their own and can keep using them for the rest of their lives.

I asked Amanda about her greatest fear at the time of this follow-up session. She responded that she was afraid that she wouldn't be as good as she was before at a job, and that if she worked too hard her condition would come back.

During the process that I shared with Amanda during this session we started with her main fears and then I allowed her subconscious to bring up related issues or memories that we cleared as we went along. Although it might seem that we were jumping from topic to topic, we were following the priority issues pushed forward by the subconscious mind that needed to be dealt with as unique issues for the complete clearing of the over-all issue.

If you are new to meridian tapping and energy therapy sessions, this process may be of interest to you and show that it is all about the emotions rather than sticking to a strict protocol or set dialog. I hope the following is helpful to you in your own fears about moving forward into the new life you are creating.

I continued to facilitate Amanda's session, and based on the weeks we had already worked together, I guided her by "putting words into her own mouth", so to speak, to set the mood even if she didn't repeat them all back to me:

> "Let's start with the **Karate Chop Point**,[61] Amanda. You can change the words I say to be your specific situation or case. You can elaborate and go beyond what I say if you want. I'm just providing the guide work for this.
>
> Even though I am afraid to move forward in my life . . .
>
> . . . I deeply and completely accept myself.
>
> Even though I really have a lot of fear about the next step in my life . . .
>
> . . . I choose to let go of that fear.
>
> I choose to see it clearly for what it is and dissolve it.
>
> I know that I can do a good job.
>
> That's a good job of healing, of staying well, and of moving forward in my life.

---

[61] For any new tappers, if you don't know where the **Karate Chop Point** is, it's on the side of the hand between the base of the little finger and the beginning of the wrist. I like to tap my two karate chop areas together.

Even though there's part of me that doesn't know if I'll be as good as I was before . . .

. . . I choose to let that go . . .

. . . because I know I'm doing the best I can do in every moment.

I know I've come a long way already.

Amanda, I want you to go back to your last job when your body was starting to fall apart. You knew you were not doing a great job for them. You knew you could have done better. You knew that the normal Amanda would have done a better job, and you knew how it felt to not get a great review and feel like you were not a good employee. On a scale of zero to ten, where are you on that?"

Amanda replied that she still felt a charge of 10 out of 10 on that... a good indication that we needed to focus some clearing at this point.

"You've got a lot of charge there. We're going to clear that. I want you to go back to thinking about how you felt back then. You knew you could do better but was your memory foggy? Were you forgetting things? I know you were absent a lot."

Amanda replied the following and mentioned that she felt a sensation in her chest:

"That was basically it because I was having chronic tonsillitis, every infection you could think of, feeling run down. I was mourning the loss of a miscarriage. I didn't get a promotion because of my absenteeism. I was going to doctors and trying to be as honest as I could. I didn't know what was wrong with me, but like clockwork every four to six weeks, I was sick with something. That's when my skin starting acting up. Perhaps that's why my skin is still acting up, because of all that resistance."

I asked her to put one hand over her chest and one hand across her forehead.

"Just go into that feeling. You lost a promotion because of your absenteeism. You were catching sickness every month. You were really worn down. You just couldn't do it anymore. Just breathe that out. If the sensation in your chest moves, follow it with your hand. You can let that go. That's heavy energy, heavy stuff. A lot of self-judgment: I should be doing a better job. They passed me up for a promotion and I really deserved it before. Now I'm absent and it's not my fault I'm getting sick all the time. I'm trying really hard. What's wrong with me? I just can't do it anymore. Just that struggle, that heavy energy of: 'My gosh, when is this going to end? What's wrong? Help!' Just let it go. Breathe it out.

Just let it go. Like going down the drain, you just can't swim your way back out of it. It just keeps getting worse and worse. 'I just can't do it anymore. What's wrong? Will I ever be able to do it again? Will I ever be able to have a memory again, to perform these tasks efficiently again? Why am I so susceptible to everything that goes by?' Just breathe it out. Let it go.

The disappointment: 'They passed me over for that promotion. I really could have gotten it and I did deserve it for who I was before I started getting sick all the time. It just doesn't seem fair. My body is sabotaging me. I know I'm a good worker. I know I deserve that promotion. I know I could do better at this job but my body is getting in the way. I can't do anything about it.' Just breathe that out. 'I feel really helpless and kind of hopeless because I think I'm going to be fired. They'll never give me a good recommendation if they do fire me. How am I ever going to get a job again?' Just breathe it out. Let it go. 'When are these symptoms going to stop showing up? It's getting worse and worse'!"

This brought the charge from a 10 down to a 5 on the 0 to 10 scale of emotional impact. She added that one of the issues still holding emotional charge was the fact that she would still have doctors' appointments on a regular basis and would have to miss work. Her fear was that she would have to explain herself again and worry that she wouldn't be believed or that her excuses wouldn't be accepted. She didn't like not being believed when her excuses were valid.

"Let's go to your **Eyebrow Points.** These are right above the nose where the hair on the eyebrow begins.[62] There's a lot of confusion there. 'How can I stay safe and keep my doctors' appointments when people may not believe that's where I'm really going or that it's all that necessary or that I have to go that often? That may sabotage my ability to get a job until I'm totally well, and even then maybe I'll still need to go for periodic checkups. Is my body going to sabotage me again just through these appointments so that nobody wants to hire me if I know I'm going to be absent on a regular basis for that?' Just breathe out any frustration or anger or impatience. 'I just want it to be over. I want to be able to move on.' Just let it go.

Now let's jump down to the **Collarbone Points**.[63] That's all about fear. I want you to go into the fear. 'Will I not be able to get hired because I tell them up front that I've got these doctors' appointments? Is that going to keep me from being a good candidate? If they ask me about my last job and why I'm no longer there and why I haven't been working, is all that information going to sabotage me? Are they going to feel like I'm too big a risk? Maybe I will get sick. Will that keep me from getting a job? If they ask me why I didn't get a good, raving review from the past job, why I didn't get that promotion, will they really believe that I was sick or will they think I just stopped working or wasn't a good worker? Will that be held against me for my next job? I want to be believed because I went through a lot of trauma. The least they can do is believe my story. Yes, I have had some fear about whether it'll come back or not. Nobody knows what will happen with my body. That's why I have to go to the

---

[62] You can use your index finger and middle finger of one hand and tap one finger on each eyebrow

[63] If you go to the base of your throat, there's a little hole there. You go down about an inch and then out about an inch on each side. I like to tap on one side with my thumb and the other side with my fingertips of the same hand.

doctors. I can get a doctor's report saying I'm ready to come back to work. Now I have a degree, so that will help me open more doors than it may have in the past. I do have a good work record. Maybe I can ask somebody from the past job if they could give me not a letter of recommendation but just a letter that I could use describing that before I got sick my work was satisfactory.'

'This goes back to my own fear. Am I going to be able to do it? Am I going to be able to hold down a fulltime job? I still have a family to take care of. I still have a young child. He's only five now and it takes a lot of energy and time in my life. Do I have time to be a mom and a wife, or do I have the energy and stamina to work fulltime with the other things going on?'

'I've thought of getting pregnant again. Where does that fit into the ratio? I know my body won't support another pregnancy if it's not well because I had a miscarriage before. However, if I'm committing to a fulltime job, is it fair to put my body through the fulltime work and regular life routine and still have that wonderful dream of getting pregnant with another child? Can I do it? Those are all things I think I want right now. Can I really do it? I don't know. Fear of the unknown. Can my body handle another pregnancy? It's gone through an awful lot since I was pregnant and lost the last baby. In the meantime, working fulltime, how many years do I have to get pregnant and hold down a fulltime job before then, and then maybe consider dropping back to part-time? Is this going to be anywhere in the ratio of my decision? I have so much to decide in my life.'

'I choose to let go of the fear that's holding me back so that I can be very conscious and clear as I make the right decisions instead of having a lot of emotion around any decision that I'm making. It's always a better decision when I can clear the emotion around it first. Then it's either logical or it's not; it's either the right thing or not. The fear of the unknown, I think I can handle it. I finished school. I'm losing weight. I'm feeling good. The symptoms are abating. Nobody knows the rest of the story. I am writing the script of my life as I go on. I just need to make sure that I'm letting go of all the heavy stuff that's been making me sick and holding me back and causing me to make emotionally-based decisions, or decisions based on past should's or other people's choices rather than my own. As I get clearer and less emotionally attached to certain things, I can know what's really best for me. I'll attract the right job and the right situation into my life so that I can be healthy and can live beyond now in a healthy, happy body.'"

Reporting that she had no emotional charge left on the issues we had just focused on, I asked Amanda to scan her last job situation and all the absenteeism and the missed promotion and how it felt to not be doing as good of a job as she really wanted to do. She mentioned at this point that she was thinking of a person with whom she had worked who had left an emotional scar with how she treated Amanda. She still was holding an 8 out of 10 charge while thinking of that person and her skeptical comments. We continued our work:

> "I want you to go back to that story and skepticism that that person had, comments she made toward you, looks she gave you. I don't know if she started any stories or made comments behind your back. Let us go to the points **Above and Below the Mouth.**[64] I want you to scan your experience with that person, feeling judged by that person, that the person really didn't believe you. Here you were struggling for your life and struggling to try to do the best job you could do, yet that person was doubting you, thought you were lying and thought you were making up symptoms or maybe that it was all in your head. She thought you were using your miscarriage as an excuse not to work. Even though she had two children of her own, you would think she'd feel some compassion, but you said her exact words were: 'I feel bad for you, but if it affects me and the work you do, then I don't feel bad for you.'
>
> Focus on how that hurt you when you heard her say that. Just breathe it out. That was her weakness and her

---

[64] You can put your index finger and middle finger horizontally right above your upper lip and below your lower lip. Tap those two points together.

ignorance. It really had nothing to do with you. She was selfishly saying: 'No matter what happens to you, it's all about me.' In a team, that's not a good attitude to have. Just breathe that out. Just let go of her energy. You've been carrying it a long time and it's unbeneficial to you. It doesn't make her change in any way for you to be carrying that all these years later."

At this point Amanda said her emotional charge on that memory had gone from an 8 to a 0 or 1. I then asked her to go back to her last job situation and asked how she felt and how she was interacting. I inquired whether there were any other individuals that caused her to feel upset emotionally. She responded:

"Probably just how the bosses were. They dragged out the whole process for the promotion for a couple of months. They mishandled it a lot. A lot of people agreed with that. They just put me through the ringer through the double interviews and the long process. The day I was told that I didn't get a promotion was from the boss's boss because she didn't want this to continue on any longer. They didn't want me to have to wait to hear what was going to be the case, but then asked me to lie to my direct boss that I didn't know. That kind of still continues to play in my head, just how they handled it. In hindsight, they both agreed they handled it wrongly, but for whatever reason that keeps playing in my head.

I think they were just really torn, and wondered if I would recover from the illness. I don't doubt for a second that they didn't care about me. They proved that after I got sick, whether it was out of their own guilt or whatever. They were really torn. I think there was different pressure. It was between me and another internal candidate, which made it harder."

I continued to facilitate while Amanda continued to tap on her meridian points for the major Central and Governing Vessel meridians... Above & Below the mouth:

"You were sitting on pins and needles. You were struggling

to do the work and really wanted the promotion. It made it harder and harder to do your work and do a good job because of all the meetings and their bad planning process. Just breathe that out and let me know when you feel that that's neutralized. They wanted the best for the company. They knew you deserved the job. They knew you were struggling. They really wanted to be able to make the right decision. Ultimately they did - because you fell apart. You couldn't have handled the promotion.

It was hard on them because they really wanted to give you the promotion. It was hard on you to be waiting and to be put through all the steps in their process. Hopefully the bosses learned a lot from the process so they won't ever do it again.

Nobody needs that kind of process, whether it's in the hiring process that you're getting ready to go through, or the promotion process, or any process. It just doesn't need to be that difficult. Breathe it out until you feel like it's shifted and it's neutral. Let it go. It's in the past. Everybody learned from it. The decision was hard for you, and it was the right decision ultimately. If they had promoted you, you might have felt guilt on top of everything else because you couldn't live up to the trust they put in you with the promotion. Just let it go. It's unbeneficial for you to be carrying that. It's okay and the next time you're up for a promotion in a healthy body where you're totally aware of how to drive your body in a conscious way, you'll get that promotion. How are you doing, Amanda?"

Amanda reported that the charge was down to a zero on that issue. So, after having worked for about an hour, I invited Amanda to go back to the original issue of moving on with her life. I asked her to gauge any resistance that she still had about moving forward, getting a good job, and going into those interviews and talking with those people. She reported that the charge was down to a 1 out of 10 and she knew she would be fine with applying for jobs and going through the interviewing process.

As I mentioned before, Amanda could serve as a good poster child for using Energy Psychology to get beyond the inner causes of some of her symptoms. She did her work and continues to work hard, although now she realizes that she can't overwork and stress herself out anymore or else she will get sick. For the first time in her life she is learning the personal balance in her life that we all have to learn.

- Veronica -

Veronica started out her session with an introduction:

> "I'm originally from Italy but I've been in Australia for five years. My condition is called **Hashimoto's.** Basically it's the immune system attacking my thyroid and destroying my thyroid. The symptoms started for me about ten years ago. I've been undernourished for a lot of time. I realized I had this condition pretty much six years ago. There are a variety of symptoms. The first and the one I'm struggling the most with is weight gain. The metabolism slows down because the thyroid can't work properly. I gained 15 to 20 kilos the first month. Then now I think I'm 35 kilos overweight. There are a lot of symptoms like fatigue and hair loss and constipation and cold sensitivity and a lot of other symptoms. The main one for me is weight gain. I did EFT back in Italy. I did something on my own. I sort of picked it up again a few months ago with a friend when we attended a workshop and I have been working with your group calls and recordings. I think EFT has helped me a lot with energy blocks and a lot of things that I want to let go of from the past. It helped me a lot with forgiveness. I think now I'm pretty much stuck. I'm pretty much sabotaging myself and finding myself in the same cycles over and over again, so I think I need some professional help."

Veronica suffered from what has been diagnosed as Hashimoto's, where the immune system attacks the thyroid. We know the thyroid is located in the neck. Anybody who's into chakras understands that the chakra in the throat is all about speaking your truth, conveying what's on your mind, speaking out against things that are done badly to you or done against you including speaking out at your abuser while being attacked or abused. If you're a little child and you've ever had an abusive parent or an angry parent or a parent that's just so overwhelmed that you find yourself walking on eggshells because you never know how the parent or caregiver is going to react, then you potentially don't feel able to share your truth. Think about any connection you might have with not being able to state your truth or feeling like you really need to say something, but you can't. That may be part of the energetic reason why the autoimmune condition could be located in your thyroid. That could have to do with Hashimoto's or Graves' disease or any kind of hypothyroidism or other thyroid issue.

Also, like in Veronica's experience, many autoimmune cases suffer fatigue, mood swings, sensitivity to cold, to hot, and hair loss. Veronica had a hair loss situation. She said it was really extreme at first. I know in my own situation with chronic fatigue and fibromyalgia, I put up with the pain, the suffering, the fatigue, the memory loss, the fuzzy thinking. But when my hair started falling out, my vanity took over and I said: "Now I've got to do something about this; this is ridiculous." We all have some of these symptoms. You know what you've suffered with and that is what I'd like you to focus on right now. Remember that this book is not just a book of other peoples' stories... it can be a therapeutic guide for you, too!

What came up for Veronica on her **Wellness Check** assessment[65] was a priority in the meridian metal category. There are two metal meridians, the lungs and the large intestine. I looked at the large intestine because that could cause a lot of her symptoms. There are two tapping points you can use for the large intestine specifically. One is taught by some EFT practitioners but it's not part of the regular protocol. It's on the **side of the upper legs** between your knee and your hip, right on the outside where your pant seam is located.

The large intestine is your colon. If you're constipated, it's all about the energy in your large intestine. The emotions that are generally held in the large intestine meridian have to do with being around people that are very controlling and that have very strong opinions or very strong moods: "This is right; this is wrong. You've got to do it my way. If I'm in this mood, you better run." It sounded like Veronica's father, who she had mentioned in her history.

She said that it was like she had to walk on eggshells her whole life. She didn't know what was going to make him angry, and was always in fear about that. She didn't know if he was going to beat her or not. She couldn't ever question him or ask if he was right. That's a thyroid issue coming from the throat chakra and speaking.

---

[65] For more information go to: http://annemerkel.com/net-wellness-check

Even though this had all happened years before, she was still carrying the stuck energy in her throat, and it also seemed to be showing up as symptoms in her large intestine and elsewhere.

Veronica had mentioned her work with forgiveness, and tapping on forgiveness is wonderful, however, if you have stored in your biofield and your subconscious mind and your limbic brain deep fear from childhood trauma, or some level of post traumatic stress, you can't forgive because you've got subconscious emotional charge still there. Until you release and clear the charge, it's still going to be there even though your mind may say: "Yes, I forgive that person. I know that person had a problem. That person had a hard childhood, too." But the part of you that's running the show, which is your subconscious and your energy field, that's keeping you alive and is aware of 95 to 98 percent of everything that's going on in your body-mind-spirit, is protecting you from getting hurt again. That part of you will not allow you to forgive, even though your left brain, your logical mind says: "Yes, I forgive, I forgive." The other side is saying: "No way, I'm not going to do that. I can't let myself be vulnerable after all that you've done to me!" That's where you have to clear, but not going in as forgiveness. We approach these issues from a different angle, and that's probably why Veronica had run into self-sabotage even after doing so much work on her own.

As I invited Veronica to tap on the Karate Chop point on the side of her hand I shared more information about the energetics of her condition.

Focusing on the large intestine addressed Veronica's constipation and potentially her weight gain issues. Irregular periods can be related to large intestine energetics, too, with the weight gain and a general sense of the metabolism being out of balance. Veronica's hormones were not being created or directed correctly by her weakened thyroid, so her body didn't know how to do what it was supposed to do.

Veronica agreed that she was feeling very out of balance. She had had a stressful childhood being in constant fear, which means that her triple warmer meridian was constantly sending out the messages to send more cortisol, send more adrenaline. It was sending stress hormones because she might need them to run away, or to fight for her life, or to freeze and hide.

That is what Veronica lived with her whole life. It became a pattern and she became addicted to the stress hormones to such an extent that the organ was having trouble secreting the hormones after many years. The other glands such as the adrenal glands maybe had to pick up the slack, but they were probably out of balance, too. When one gland goes out of balance, all of the others are also because they work in balance with each other. That's why if you've got an overactive thyroid, you probably have an underactive adrenal. If you have an overactive or depleted adrenal, it's just the opposite, the thyroid then will be underactive. It's all about rebalancing.

In Veronica's case, she grew up with lots of stress and it continued. She grew up in Italy, then she got married. She was shocked when she found out she was pregnant with her first child, and she moved to Australia soon after that.

Anybody that has moved from one culture to another, or has had an early childhood with a lot of stress in it is going to find things like a move from one culture to another to be quite a big stress. Even if you're very organized and have it under control, it can be stressful for your system. Veronica was excited about the move, but she was still stressed... and that was added to an already stressed-out system.

On a certain level, Veronica's body was already weakened because of the stress of her early childhood. Then she added a very happy move to it, but all the details of a move, moving from one climate to another, language changes, culture changes, her husband had a new assignment in his job, the baby had to change schools. All that is stressful, even though in a good way. I felt that this was what had gotten Veronica close to the point where she had been diagnosed with Hashimoto's, but there was still that "final straw" or situation that pushed her over the edge.

There's always one thing that brings all the rest of the stress to a head. That's why they say you've got a camel with lots of straw on its back. You put on one more tiny, little piece of straw, and the camel collapses. The "last straw" on Veronica's camel came when she was working a stressful job because her then-partner but now husband was not getting a salary. She was earning the money for her family, and that was very stressful. There was a lot of responsibility on her back then, and she collapsed into a diagnosed illness with lots of symptoms.

The question now was how to rebalance. The tapping would support her body to get better and to rebalance itself.

During our tapping sequence together we covered Veronica's following issues clearing emotional baggage or charge from each of them:

- "Dad stressed me out and was unpredictable, angry, abusive, and irrational."
- "I lived a stressful hyper vigilant life that I learned to survive living with my dad."
- "My life was unsafe for my body."
- "I am angry at dad for his child abuse... it is inexcusable!"
- "I felt unloved by my parents."
- "My best never seemed good enough for you."
- "Nobody ever praised me for being a good girl."
- "My mother never wanted me, and even told me that."
- "Mom never loved me."
- "I am surrounded now by love."
- "I love myself and choose to become healthy!"

I have provided Veronica's tapping sequence for you later in this book.[66]

At the end of her session Veronica reported:

> "I feel so much calmer. I feel like – I'm smiling and I don't know even why. I feel great."

Even though Veronica has more issues around which to tap, by working with a facilitator we were able to together clear the deeper aspects of root cause issues in her life so that she can work on day-to-day and less life-impacting issues on her own. I like to say that

---

[66] Check out *Tapping Sequence 7*.

I'll help clear the large boulders while you can take care of the rocks and pebbles along your life path.

More Therapeutic Tools to Remember

Before I end this section on Veronica, I'd like to share and remind you of some special tools that you can use for emotional issues like we discussed in this case or for cases of trauma and anxiety. These can be added to your regular meridian tapping or EFT practice.

Remember that if you've got a **Large Intestine** issue, or even if you don't, it's a good thing to add the leg tapping position into your regular EFT tapping protocol. It's a very important meridian to use whether you tap or rub that outside of your leg between the hip and knee.

Another helpful large intestine tapping point is on the base of the index finger nail. This is a traditional EFT hand tapping point, and I find that you can actually tap on the index finger nail base using either the same hand thumb or middle finger. This can be very therapeutic, and it stimulates the end acupuncture point of the meridian.

Another large intestine place that you can use is on your face. Pretend that you're getting ready to jump into a lake or swimming pool and you're going to hold your nose shut so you don't take in water through your nose. In doing this you'll start to pinch your nostrils with your thumb and index finger. Do that and gently un-pinch, bring your fingers away so you're not touching your nose but you're almost touching it, and from this position tap gently on your cheeks right there on the edge of either side of each nostril. If you've got a head cold and you're constipated, by tapping here, sometimes you can feel some big sinus shifts. That can actually ease constipation just by tapping there. If you're constipated, your sinuses are often blocked, too. You may have symptoms of a cold until you actually eliminate and then your cold symptoms disappear, which shows that you never had a cold; those were just the symptoms that your large intestine was blocked. You can unblock the energies involved in the meridians by tapping the large intestine meridian as it passes through your sinuses.

Another exercise I definitely want to teach you before we end here is how to cross your arms therapeutically to turn down the **Triple Warmer** meridian which stimulates production of the stress hormones, and to raise the energy in the **Spleen** meridian that enhances your self-esteem. It's a simple thing that can not only protect your energy field, which runs up the front of your body, but can also help to balance your personal power center around your **Third Chakra** at the solar plexus, right above your navel and below your ribcage.

The way to cross your arms for extra meridian balance is to take one arm, either one, and put it across your body, just like you're crossing your arms, but with this hand you're going to touch the **Under Arm** tapping point, right where a woman's bra strap would be, with your fingers. You'll touch your fingers there and then kind of cup your breast with the rest of your hand. The spleen meridian is what you're holding or tapping on via the **Under Arm Point**. Then the meridian continues under your breast. You're going to have your hand touching that. Next, place your other arm over the top of the first arm, and grab the back of your lower arm just above the elbow with the fingers of the upper arm. With the bottom hand you're touching the **spleen meridian**, which is the Under Arm tapping point and under your breast. The upper arm is the **triple warmer meridian**. That is the meridian that's in charge of all the stress hormones and from the limbic or unconscious brain, it sends hormones with the messages: "You've got to fight. You've got to run. You've got to freeze!" If you just hold that position for a short while, you'll find that it's very calming. When you feel tired of that position, just shift arms and put the top arm on the bottom and the bottom arm on the top.

This is a wonderful exercise if you grew up being hyper vigilant where you were always in constant fear or always on guard. Anyone with this condition has lived constantly with underlying stress in their body. This cross-the-arms technique is a perfect tool that can be utilized anytime you're sitting around, where you can automatically balance those two meridians to turn down the stress hormones and turn up the sense of self-esteem and presence.

I think many of us living in Western Society could use all of these tools... especially the last one! Try them all on yourself!

- Helen -

Helen's case was a classic for the Metal Element meridians of the Lung and Large Intestine. Her life had some of the same themes as Veronica's case. At 23 years she presented to me with serious hives, eczema, psoriasis and a long list of life traumas. Helen had felt suicidal several times and had felt like she could not escape from a life in which she was a victim.

I liked this young lady's spunk. She had a great sense of humor and playful spirit, and I hoped that I could help her to find that joy for which she had been searching her whole life.

Because she felt so hopeless and helpless before finding EFT Tapping, the shifts in her attitude as a result of meridian tapping helped her to find me and initiate a month of weekly sessions.

The Wellness Check showed her Metal meridians way out of balance, along with other layers of anger, but I realized from her extensive history that she the Lung and Large Intestine were the areas where we would focus most of our work together.

The Metal Profile

When I work with clients who present with skin issues I normally look for Metal meridians, and in Helen's case her life was surrounded by Metal issues.

In traditional Chinese acupuncture there are five elements and each contains certain meridians. In this system as well as some western systems such as NET/ Neuro Emotional Technique, in which I am trained, various meridians and specific points generally correlate with different physical or emotional issues.

- According to NET, the **Lung meridian** generally relates to Grief and often a sense of Loss. It also sometimes may relate to the following: Sadness, yearning, cloudy thinking, and anguish.

- Using that same NET system, the **Large Intestine meridian** generally relates to the energy of being

"Dogmatically positioned" or very controlling or set in one's opinions or ways of living life. It also sometimes may relate to the following: Crying, compelled to neatness, defensive.

- Where my experience is that the **Lung** energy of loss is most often first hand, the heavy controlling and "my mind is set" energy of the **Large Intestine** can be the individual or someone else in that person's life whose heavy-handed influence has tended to thwart his or her personal power of choice in life.

When Helen first contacted me to be a "test subject" in my autoimmune studies, her approach was very forthright and clear. She really wanted to work with me and was willing to stick her neck out to be noticed. She told me that prior to her tapping experience of almost a year before we met, she was timid and did not speak up for herself. She attributed the meridian tapping to her new-found ability to ask for what she needed, and I saw this as a good sign as she was beginning to create the life she desired for the first time in her life.

Helen's History

Helen was an intelligent multi-lingual, multi-cultural young lady with parents from two different cultures. Her parents had met when they both were globe-trotting professionals, and in the course of their early marriage her mother got pregnant. This was not good news, as her mother traveled internationally with her corporation for months at a time and loved her career. Before getting married her mom had believed her suitor to be much more of a gentleman than the man she found herself married to. She was about to leave this violent man when she found she was pregnant. Believing she had been set up by her husband, she felt trapped into becoming a mother. Soon after Helen was born her mom resumed her travels and so the baby was left with the violent, moody, controlling father and an absent mother who might be gone for several months and then return for several days up to a couple of weeks before taking off again. Poor little Helen growing up never knew when her mother would be there for her or when she would be deserting her again. She felt like she had lost her mother from the time of her conception because it was made clear to her that she was not wanted by her mom... who already felt trapped and controlled in the role of motherhood. So began the recurring negative patterns of feeling trapped and out of control as well as being abandoned over and over. These both could have led to Helen's early development of serious asthmatic lung issues and then later the serious skin issues.

At the age of 8 years old Helen was taken from her happy life in her home country where she had friends, loved to play outside in the temperate climate, and where the language and customs were familiar to her. She was uprooted and taken to her father's country without any say-so or seeming regard for the total inconvenience to a little girl living with a difficult man and no mother. A few weeks after arriving Helen suffered a life-threatening asthma attack that landed her in the hospital on a ventilator for two weeks. The new environment was unfriendly, dark, cold and rainy, and the culture seemed unfriendly to her. Her remark was that she had always felt suffocated by her family, and living alone with her dad in this unfamiliar culture left her feeling "suffocated to death" as she stated.

Helen had always excelled in school subjects and under the control of her dad even her grades began to drop when he showed little regard for her desire to study for exams or to initiate anything that might push her own life ahead. It almost seemed to her that her dad looked down his nose at her and wanted her to fail. Even her teachers were shocked at her lackluster end-of-term exam scores, knowing she could have done much better. But dad had insisted that she go out with her cousins rather than study for the exams, so she did well but did not excel. She said there was and still is a part of her that is afraid to disagree with her father.

At sixteen years Helen said she suffered a serious trauma when her father didn't let her choose her upper high school subjects. She was sent to a school she did not choose, to study courses she didn't like, and ended up trying to change subjects until she was stuck for two years in a curriculum that she hated and in which she didn't care to make good grades. She hated being tagged an "unstable and unreliable teen". This was the start of what she calls her "suicidal phase", and just points out how she felt unrecognized for who she was and totally unheard.

After two years she graduated and ran away back to her country of birth to "escape her father". She said that from then on her life was filled with trauma after trauma. She tried to enter the university there but they were ahead of her and there was a language issue. She suffered a traumatic break-up from a boyfriend, and then somehow got metal poisoning from which she almost died, that led to the Eczema/ Psoriasis outbreak from which she still suffered. At that point her mother demanded that she go back to her father's country and enroll there in the university.

At age 21 Helen went to university and wasn't enjoying the courses chosen for her. Her parents were finally getting a divorce and she was excited that this might mean freedom not only for her mother but for her too. She had an opportunity to start special courses in the major of her desires but her parents shocked her when they both insisted that she stay in her current studies at the same institution, and the light of freedom was quickly extinguished. She turned down her opportunity and later dropped out of university and had been working at low income jobs since then. Around this time she developed open sore hives that were her main complaint when she presented to me.

Helen has suffered from the following "Metal" issues among others:
- Loss of mother's acceptance and love,
- Loss of the presence of her mother,
- Loss of her childhood homeland and her early "persona",
- Loss of self-esteem around grades and personal accomplishments,
- Loss of freedom to make her own decisions,
- Subject to control and volatility of father,
- Subject to decisions of parents (sounds like most children or young adults),
- Loss of sense of "Self" and freedom of choice.

Some of her physical symptoms which all fit into the "Metal" category:
- Breathing issues,
- Skin issues: Eczema/ Psoriasis from control & loss,
- Skin issues: Intense Hives from anxiety and fear of father,
- Deep skin sensitivities based on lack of control of her life.

After we worked together Helen was reporting that she felt calmer, her skin was much better, she was able to feel hope again, and was spending more quality time with her mother.

She planned to go back to school in the field she had chosen and was continuing to clear her emotional issues using EFT tapping on her own. She was also working with an acupuncturist who had a good reputation, so she was hopeful that many of her body-mind-spirit issues would resolve.

I have included the tapping sequence[67] that we used for her first session in the back of this book in case you resonate with the issues listed here and would like to use her tapping sequence as a guide. Just change the words and issues as you let it lead you with the points to tap as well as the types of comments you can make with the tapping sequence.

More Therapeutic Tools - from Energy Medicine

As I began working with Helen I wanted to give her a daily routine and help her to access her body's inner energy, subconscious, and provide more clarity in her life. I shared with her Donna Eden's "Four Thumps"[68] morning protocol and I also showed her how to cross her arms to balance the Spleen and Triple Warmer meridians[69] whenever she felt anxious.

The **"Four Thumps"** is a wonderful exercise to use first thing in the morning. This exercise includes "thumping" rather than tapping on four meridian energy points:
- EFT *Collarbone Points* = K27 points
- *Thymus Point* in the center of the upper chest.
- EFT *Spleen Points*
- EFT *Under Eye Points*

Before we got started in sessions I wanted to get Helen engaged energetically. We got centered, connected our energies, and called

---

[67] See Tapping Sequence 8.
[68] Eden, Donna, with Feinstein, D., PhD (2008) Energy Medicine: Balancing Your Body's Energies for Optimal Health, Joy, and Vitality. New York, NY: Penguin Group Publishers.
[69] I shared this in the previous chapter under "Therapeutic Tools to Remember".

in our Divine Helpers. Then we enthusiastically "thumped" the above points until we each felt enlivened and ready to get into the clearing of the session. I highly recommend using this tool in your own life.

- Kristen -

Kristen's initial case revolved around her skin issues from which she had suffered for four years following the seeming total collapse of a life fraught with trauma and loss.

Kristen's History

When Kristen's legs and back broke out with open sores and itchiness she was diagnosed with Chronic Demylinating Polyneuropathy with genetic mutation of the methylenetetrahydrofolate gene. [70] [71]

Three years after this diagnosis Kristen found me and we started working together to clear some of her underlying pain. She was already aware of and using EFT tapping when we met, and she realized she needed an experienced facilitator to guide her path.

Kristen reported that the overall tone of her early life was conflict, fighting, walking on eggshells, pretending to be outside of the house, wishing she lived in another family.

Looking over her history a number of issues popped out at me including:
- Fourth child – was supposed to be a son, finally – wasn't... but was treated well as youngest child by father – mother didn't want any more children,
- Sickly child – traumatized by doctor administering shots
- Watched father physically & emotionally abusing oldest brother
- Age 7: Tonsillectomy – left alone in hospital

---

[70] Science now has proven in the field of epigenetics that genes can change based on the whole environment of an organism, and for Kristen, that environment was one of stress, abuse, loss, trauma, more abuse, and more trauma... all creating toxic emotional environments conducive to genetic shifts... for survival.

[71] Further specific research relating to Kristen's experience is the Polyvagal Theory pointing out how phylogenetic change occurs in certain cases of extreme trauma or stress based on the regulation of the vagus nerve in its earlier and later adaptations. For more information on this theory by Dr. Stephen Porges, see **Appendix 3** in this book.

- Age 5-40: Elder sister physically & emotionally abusive
- Age 7.5: Last sibling born - a son – she went from being "baby of family to 'nothing' of family"
- Age 8: Older brother hit by car – in serious condition
- Age 15: Mother raged – tore up her room, hit her, cut her arm with a knife sending her to hospital saying it was an accident, etc.
- Age 17: She ran away from home to another state where a sister with whom she was close lived – her dad came to take her home – during the conversation urging her to join him on his flight home he promised that if her mom didn't get psychiatric help she could stay with her sister and finish school there.
- She left with her dad, preferring to take a bus, but he insisted on the plane ride – their plane crashed, killing her father and leaving her in the hospital for a month following a Near-Death out-of-body experience.[72]
- After arriving home her mother tells her she killed her father and to GET OUT before she kills everyone else. Kristen shut down inside.
- 4 months after crash: she gets pregnant – marries father of her son – not in love.
- ~ Age 25-6: her husband is busted for pot – she was left alone with her son, but could not connect as a mom.
- Later 20's: ran away from life – partying – just couldn't connect – her son left with his father's parents.
- Married briefly & divorced – he was an alcoholic and committed suicide.
- Age 27: Started ten years of therapy.
- Age 28: Lost a year then hooked up with a doctor – married – tubal pregnancy killing her chances of any more children – husband having an affair – divorced after 5 years at age 32.
- Age 38: met her next husband.
- Age 41: Married for 3 years – divorced due to his 900 sexual

---

[72] An event as traumatic as a plane crash often triggers the most ancient aspect of the vagus nerve, which serves to shut down the system and lead to phylogenetic changes within the survivor. See **Appendix 3** or go to: Porges, Stephen W., PhD. (2011) **The Polyvagal Theory: Neurophysiological Foundations of Emotions, Attachment, Communication, and Self-regulation** (Norton Series on Interpersonal Neurobiology). New York: NY/ Norton & Co., Inc.

abuse and alcoholism issues. She "was DONE and severely heart-broken".

- Age 44: mother has heart attack in her car – dies days later. Horrible time with family members.
- Age 45: moved to California from the NE USA to start 3 years of self-healing.
- Age 41-55: in relationship with another "loser".
- Age 55-59: She flies her ailing eldest brother to CA from FL to help him. Nobody else to care for him after he lost his leg to diabetes, non-care, alcohol. Took him into her home to care for him, then set him up in an apartment. Led to deep grief, deep loss, and deep anger when he turned against her in his last days, called in his ex-wife and daughter plus their older abusive sister, who took Kristen's belongings from the apartment and excluded her from his death process after all she had done for him. They seemed to want credit for taking care of him... for weeks instead of years, like Kristen.
- Age 57: Financially struggling and almost loses her home because of debt paying for brother's care. Her lease on business space ends so she must move business elsewhere. Tax issues arise with large attorney fees.
- Age 59: Brother dies.
- Age 60: Rash begins.
- Age 60-63: very sick, exhausted, severe rashes, severe itching, some infections, swelling, using 8 physicians both allopathic & alternative, plus acupuncture, colonics, infusions, IV antibiotics, nerve testing, hyperbaric oxygen chamber, plus meds, vitamins, and beginning to EFT tap.

Like so many of my other clients, Kristen didn't want to live a life stuck in this old pattern of suffering. She was seeking a way out, so we started our energy therapy work together.

After just one month of weekly calls the painful lesions and rash on her legs were clearing to the extent that she could start wearing clothes more appropriate for warmer summer days. See Kristen's dramatic "before" and "after" leg photos in **Appendix 4** at the end of this book.[73]

---

[73] In addition to viewing the distinct difference in her leg lesions after four sessions using energy psychology added to her on-going health protocol, **Appendix 4** also lists the issues that we covered in her sessions.

Focus on Moving Forward

Kristen and I began our work in mid-January. We cleared early life issues first and saw some dramatic physical results. We continued to work on issues that came up or were triggered in Kristen's life as well as their related deeper root cause issues.

By mid-March, just after a session where we had cleared Kristen's issues of "safety" in her life, she came to me with big news.

In just two months Kristen had gone from being a fearful, unhealthy, emotionally-damaged 63-year-old to now deciding that she was going to close her service business location 25 miles from her home and was going to move her practice, livelihood, and full client base to her own town to work under the umbrella of another business. She had already started looking at spaces and interviewing commercial land-lords. She had a friend working on her PR announcements, and she was looking into special incentives for her clients to drive the 25 miles to her, instead of her needing to drive to them. She had a vision and she was already moving forward on it!

This was exciting news, and it brought up some distinct advantages to her lifestyle as well as stressful issues. The benefits were no more commute, and in fact, she bought a bicycle to ride to work on nice days. She also would be paying much less in monthly commercial space rental. Stressful issues she would have to face included those of change, loss of owning her own business, fear of losing clients, trust in working with others, communication, disappointment when a couple of nice spaces fell through, among other themes that we cleared together in the next few weeks as they came up.

Even though Kristen realized that this change – letting go of a wonderful former location working for herself with employees, potentially losing some old clients, and re-creating her practice in a new location with new management, new environment, and new colleagues - would create stress in her life, her body dealt with it by producing one deep leg lesion that became infected so required that she visit her doctor for antibiotics. She monitored her stress, and other than this, she used her meridian tapping successfully, continued to stay on a paleo-type diet[74], and got exercise and more sleep since she didn't have to commute after the move of her business.

During this time of transition we had a session that helped her to clear out her visceral nervousness and reactions to the change going on all around her.

Kristen's Session

I asked Kristen to describe what was going on during the months leading up to this point in her life:

> "First of all, I had no energy. I was using any chance I could get to take a nap when I wasn't working – I'm not talking 15 minutes, I'm talking a couple hour naps. Sometimes they were three hours long, plus sleeping at night. I was completely exhausted. I had to change my entire way of eating. I totally gave up dairy and grains. I pretty much eat a Paleo diet. Sugar, caffeine – I'm not a soda drinker or anything like that. I had to give up all of that stuff. I also had to give up socializing a lot because I just couldn't – people would invite me to do things. I would think: 'Okay, I can go.' The time would come and I just wouldn't have the energy. I only had the energy to take care of myself and to go to work, because I'm self-employed and I'm single and I own a home. Those are the only things that I was capable to take care of. And see the doctors and all that, try to get well.
>
> I made a big decision, when the lease was up this year, to move my salon from a town 25 miles away to the town where I live, which will save me a lot of money and a lot of time. I'll be closer to home, and be able to have my life be much more simplified. I have been a salon owner since 1984. This is a big change for me.
>
> I've had great luck with my clients, believe it or not. Thank

---

[74] For more information go to: Ballantyne, S., PhD. (2013) **The Paleo Approach: Reverse Autoimmune Disease and Heal Your Body.** USA: Victory Belt Publishing.

you, Archangel Michael,[75] who has been right there hanging in. They're all happy to come. They all get why I'm doing this. I'm being supported."

I continued to facilitate the session:

"I want to invite you, Kristen, to go to your upper chest, above the breast area and under the collarbones. Feel around in your upper chest to see if you've got any area there that might be a little tender. You've got neurolymphatic points all over your upper chest where you can feel tenderness sometimes when you're holding emotions, are stressed out about something like change in your life, or have some subconscious resistance.

If you feel a sore spot in your upper chest, I want you to massage it. It may be real tender, but as you massage it, it will stop being tender. As you're doing that, I want you to think about what inner resistance you have about change. What are you not allowing yourself to let go of? What kind of stress are you feeling because of some of the things in your life that are changing? They might be out of your control. Maybe you don't have the memory you used to. Maybe you're having physical symptoms that are just not seeming healthy and not something you want to have in or on your body, but they're there. Things out of your control may be causing stress. A lot of change is out of our control while even some of the change that we are controlling can also be stressful. Focus on what's going on in your life, whether you like it or not, and how that feels as you're massaging any sore areas in your upper chest.

Breathe out the soreness as you also breathe out that stress or inner resistance that you may be feeling. You're moving forward with changes. You can't go back. I always tell

---

[75] Kristen has a deep Spiritual belief – especially since her Near-death experience during the plane crash. She works regularly with her diseased sister as well as Archangels Michael and Raphael. They give her support and she delegates special tasks to them with the faith that they will carry through in ways that she'd never be able to manage. She continues to be grateful for their support.

people that autoimmune is not a life sentence of suffering. It is, however, a life sentence of being aware and of diligently being responsible for your body, mind, and spirit. It's not just life as usual. It's different. You don't fit in with the masses of the general population. You can't eat what they eat. You can't do what they do to the same extent. For some of us, it is an enlightenment situation where we learn that we didn't enjoy doing some of that stuff anyway. The new lifestyles that we create can be so much less stressful and more rewarding and can truly empower each of us to really be more of who we really are instead of wearing a mask to work or wearing a mask in a relationship, or just wearing a mask and not truly being ourselves and enjoying who we are.

Let's move to the **Karate Chop Point**, right at the base of the little finger on the flat side of the hand. I'd like you to tap there. Feel a sense of gratitude for this beautiful body that you have that is so much smarter than we'll ever be. Do you know that your logical left brain mind only knows about two percent of what's going on? Yet we give it all the power to try to solve all the problems. We give it the power to worry or to rationalize one way or the other. It doesn't know what the body knows. It doesn't know what the energy system knows. It doesn't know what the emotional subconscious mind knows. It doesn't know what your great grandparents and your parents and all your ancestors suffered through and that you inherited in your DNA. It didn't know what kind of stress your mother had when she was pregnant with you, and what kind of stress you incurred in the birthing process, which is a very stressful process for any baby.

Your logical mind doesn't know what kind of beliefs and comments and innuendos and emotional tone was fed to you from the time you were born up until age ten or twelve when your cognitive mind started to really notice that you were separate from your primary care givers. You don't know all the data that you were fed, all the bad looks, all the potential things that people said in judgment of you that your subconscious took in and accepted as true. You don't remember feeling other people's stress around you when you were very young related to change of any kind. Your subconscious is like a sponge. It takes on anybody else's feelings that you feel along with them. If you can relate, then it becomes part of your own subconscious. Your logical mind doesn't know what's in there. That's why we need to connect with the energy system through tapping and other ways, like rubbing the **Sore Spots**, to help the subconscious mind let go of the stuff that we don't know about, all the old patterns, the old history, the things we've forgotten or we've stuffed, the scary movies we watched when we were young. We believed them on some level to be true. Stories of other people's tragedies that we took on will affect us until we clear them.

Change can be real scary, even good change. Look at your body. Your body is going through changes or else you wouldn't be on this call. Some of the changes are scary. The big words that you get from the practitioners that you go to and their diagnosis, the treatment, the prognosis, so many practitioners coming from Western medicine believe truly, because this is what they're taught, that there is no cure for autoimmune disorders. Some will tell you it's just in your mind. Nothing is really showing up on any of the tests. It's really not in your body, you're just imagining this, so you must be crazy. Other people tell you to go home and learn to live with it. Those kinds of information are horrible to take on.

I want you to think now about any time that anybody has told you about something like that. I want you to move your tapping to right **Under the Eye**. There's a bone there that is the edge of the eye socket bone. Tap right on the little edge there under your eye and think back to any bad news that you got from a doctor or a health practitioner or anybody who didn't believe your story, didn't believe your pain, treated you in a way that was uncomfortable to you, thought they could help you but the drugs didn't work or the treatment didn't work or the protocol didn't work. Focus on times when maybe you've done tapping and you haven't felt immediate results and you felt really disappointed and let down. I want you to just think about anything that people told you about your suffering that you didn't feel like you could accept, or that you just felt like what they said was not correct, you could not relate to it. Let's just breathe that out. That causes a lot of stress that you do not need to be carrying!

Any kind of change, whether you're looking at your body and noticing symptoms or changes, or you are focusing on the change in progress of shifting your life for the good out of necessity or choice. Let's go to the points right at the base of your neck. Tap now on the **Collarbone Point.** I like to tap with my thumb on one side and my fingertips on the other side. This is all about fear. Being diagnosed with an autoimmune condition can bring up a lot of fear. And then being told that you have to change the way you're living, change your lifestyle, change what you wear because you might want to cover up something that's breaking out on your body somewhere. You may have to limit how often you go out to eat, whether it's to somebody else's house or to a restaurant because you can't eat the same foods you used to be able to eat. You may feel like you're becoming really high maintenance so you'd rather just stay home and cook for yourself. But maybe that's not who you used to be. Maybe you're really an extrovert and you really like social encounters and this is cramping your style.

There can be a lot of fear about change of any kind. It could be fear that you're never going to get well even if you do make lifestyle changes. You may be afraid that if you make these lifestyle changes for your health condition that other people aren't going to be around you. They're not going to want to stay with you. They're not going to want to watch you go through this, or they're not going to want to go where you are. You may be afraid that they're going to want somebody that has more vitality like you used to have. Just breathe out any fear of loss – real or perceived."

Kristen gave her perception on this:

"What it has been like for me has been finally understanding the truth of what happened and being validated about it. That's been amazing to me. It hasn't been like going into the pain of it again, but it has been an understanding and completing of something that had never been completed in my life. The fear and trauma just stayed stuck in my body. As we talked and tapped through the stories of my life the subconscious started to understand the rest of the story and fear disappeared."

I continued:

"Let's go on to the **Under Arm Point**. That's all about self-esteem and finding your courage and amping it up. You have the ability to move forward even though change is necessary, including some controlled change, some planned change, some intentional change, and some uncontrolled change, but you do have that ability to go through the change without heightened stress. You also have the ability to clear stress around change as you feel it. That is the best time to tap away the stress, when you're feeling it.

Just breathe out the stress. Breathe in a sense of wellbeing and courage to move forward. Again, breathe out any feelings of limitation. Most of your limitation is based on fear, which is false evidence appearing real, FEAR. You believe it on some level and you can clear that and let it go. Go back into the true essence of who you are. We are all powerful, creative beings. Yes, we can clear the causes of why we're sick. We can move forward and create a wonderful new life just like you're doing, Kristen. Just breathe out all the old resistance and blocks. Let go of that fear about moving forward. Moving forward is a wonderful opportunity that can bring so much joy and personal power and satisfaction and new things that you've never ever experienced in your life. Focus on how it's going to feel when we get the results. Then let God or the Universe or your helpers or angels come up with the details. They'll be so much better than anything you could ever plan. You just have to get out of the way and let go of all resistance to change and fear about change. Then you will get your reward.

Let's go up to the **Top of Head** now. Use your fingertips and just move it around and tap the top of your head. As you're doing that, I want you to feel gratitude, gratitude that there really is hope that you can get well and that you can create a wonderful life on your terms that's healthy, that allows you to have energy and fun and experience love and peace of mind for the rest of your life. There are tools that are easy to use that you can use whenever you need them. And so it is.

Just breathe out the stress. You can stop tapping now. Breathe in a deep breath of peace of mind. Feel it coming in and just totally filling you up. Now breathe out all the old stuff, all the frustration, the old stuff that's been keeping you stuck or resisting or just not feeling like you can go forward. Just breathe that out. Take one more big breath and breathe in the energy of opportunity. All the wonderful things in the universe that are right there for us but we have blinders on. Breathe out the blinders. Let go of all your limitations. Just let them go. All they do is hold you back and limit your life and limit your perspective. Now take a big drink of water."

At the end of this short session Kristen reported that she felt lighter and calmer, and especially while tapping at the **Collar Bone** for fear she felt a lot of shifting and feeling in her stomach. She was not as nervous as before.

Any move is stressful, and even good change can cause stress to an already-stressed system. All in all Kristen came through this with flying colors and after several set-backs and then remodeling time for the new space, she opened her business on time and was delighted to discover that most of her clients were happy to follow her to the new location.

Kristen and I stay in contact, and she continues to move forward into areas which felt blocked to her for much of her life. We plan to get into some deeper work regarding the plane crash and the vagus nerve issues[76] that may still be causing some underlying anxiety. In the meantime, she is tapping away daily stressors and asks for help

---

[76] See **Appendices 3 & 4**.

when new changes come into her life. At the rate she is now living her life, major shifts continue to happen regularly and she now has more energy to put into these so that she can reap the benefits of the life she is creating!

Tapping Sequences

Often people first learning to use meridian tapping modalities such as EFT on their own don't know how to create their own scripts to guide their tapping sequences. Having a facilitator often helps considerably.

Gerry remarked, as well as others, how much more profound the tapping became when the main focus was not just on the words spoken, but on the emotions felt as the words brought up memories, issues, old wounds.

As a facilitator I strive to keep my client in the emotional energy or right brain subconscious feeling sense unless they suffer acute PTSD/ post traumatic stress disorder. In our sessions I ask the client to repeat after me so that they can feel and hear the words describing the feeling as they tap on a specific point.

As a facilitator of several different meridian tapping modalities, I find that it is advantageous to focus energy at each point before going to the next one, so instead of making one phrase or statement per point and moving to the next, we focus on clearing various aspects of an issue held at a specific tapping point before going on. (This "N-hanced EFT" process gets even more specific correlating specific emotions to tapping points in the 2014-15 cases after Gerry's case.) So, one tapping sequence of N-hanced EFT may include one full round of EFT tapping points or may jump around and only use certain points according to the emotions coming up.

If you relate to one of the issues described in a case within this book, it might behoove you to try tapping along with the script as you focus on your own "story".

And, if you are not yet acquainted with EFT or the tapping point locations, you may access my complimentary training package.[77]

---

[77] Sign up at: http://annemerkel.com/free-eft-stuff/

Tapping Sequence 1 –

Gerry & Her Values

After Gerry completed the **Values Assessment Exercise**[78], she realized that in her own mind she had resistance to being healthy in her body, mind, spirit. On a scale of 10 items she placed her Health as #5 until after we cleared her inner blocks using this and the following meridian tapping sequences.

At some point in her life she had lost faith in everyone around her, including God, and so her body, which had been physically abused during her early life, became something that she began to feel also was abusing her or giving her what she felt she deserved. In this session she gave her body permission to heal and started realizing that she could accept this as a high priority.

"Start tapping the **Karate Chop point**:

Even though part of me wants to stay the way I am right now . . .
. . . I deeply and completely accept myself.

I accept that I am doing my best at where I am right now.

I accept that this belief that I'm where I need to be may change.

Even though part of me believes I need to keep this illness in my body . . .
. . . or I deserve to live with this in my body right now . . .
. . . I deeply and completely accept myself . . .
. . . and I accept that this can change.

Edge of the Eyebrow point:

In the past, I have felt unworthy.

---

[78] This can be found at: http://annemerkel.com/free-eft-stuff/

In the past, I have felt that I deserved to be ill.

In the past, I have felt like a victim.

In the past, I have felt very confused.

In the past, I have felt like the whole world was assaulting me.

I felt like I deserved to be assaulted by the world.

Everything that would come in my direction, pollen or smoke or perfume, was an assault on me.

I accepted that.

I became a victim of that.

I really believed that that was the role I was to play.

I played it for a long time.

Now it's time to change.

I am ready to let go of the anger I have about that.

I have been really angry that I have given myself this sentence of ill health.

I am angry that I have given myself this ill health.

I choose to let it go now.

Outside of Eye point:

I resent all of the assaults I've had in my life.

Even when I do this tapping work, I feel assaulted.

I feel like a victim.

I don't know if I feel like a victim when I do the tapping.

It brings up old victim memories.

I choose to let go of this feeling.

I choose to let go of the confusion I have felt.

I choose to allow myself to heal.

It's time for this body to heal.

I'm ready to do different things in my life.

I'm ready to let go of the mentality of an infant.

Even though I was treated badly as an infant and young child . . . and later at my job, I happened to be in the presence of some toxic materials . . .
. . . I can still overcome this and let go of ever being a victim.

I can heal from all of these wounds.

I choose to heal from all of these wounds.

I deserve to heal from all of these wounds.

I want to heal from all of these wounds.

My Highest Self wants me to heal from all of these wounds.

The Universe wants me to heal from all of these wounds.

God wants me to heal from all of these wounds.

The people that abused me felt so ashamed that they want me to heal all these wounds.

It's time for me to heal now.

Underneath the Eye:

As I look back at the traumas I have experienced . . .

I feel really disgusted.

I feel really angry.

I've held these feelings a long time.

It's time for me to let go of them now.

These feelings serve nobody.

For me to be the best human being I can be . . .
. . . it's time for me to let go of these old beliefs that are keeping my body sick.

Tap with *two fingers Above and Below the mouth:*

When I was abused as an infant and small child, I felt unworthy of anything better.

I felt that this is what I deserved.

I felt that a good, easy life was un-deserved by me.

I was supposed to suffer.

I was supposed to have pain in my body.

I was supposed to be slowed down so I couldn't speak my truth.

I was supposed to be held back so that I couldn't really be the true me that I wanted to be.

I was controlled by others.

All of this felt really horrible.

This made me feel that I was worthless.

This made me feel that I should suffer.

This made me feel that I deserved a life of suffering.

This made me feel that I really deserved to be assaulted all the time in my life.

I became very sensitive.

I have taken on many things from others and from the environment that have affected my body and my emotions.

It's time for me to get well and to heal.

This suffering has gone on long enough.

I choose to heal now.

I know I can heal as I let go of these old beliefs.

These beliefs are negative and detrimental to me.

I deserve better.

I want me to heal.

Everybody wants me to heal.

It's time for me to let go of everything that's holding me back.

I choose to let go of the fatigue.

I choose to let go of the toxins.

I choose to let go of the old beliefs that I deserve to suffer.

Collarbone point:

I'm afraid of who I will be without the suffering.

I'm terrified of who I will be without -- it will be so unfamiliar without all this suffering.

What kind of a person will I turn into without all these aches and pains and fatigue?

What kind of a person will I turn into without all this fatigue?

Then I'll have to grow up and shoulder some responsibility and take my life on again.

This is scary.

I haven't done it for years because I've been working on healing my body . . .
. . . or I've been living with the fatigue and stress so I haven't been able to take on the responsibility.

Now if my body heals and my energy comes back, then what am I going to do?

Do I have what it takes to live a life without this pain?

Do I have what it takes to live without this fatigue and emotional pain?

Am I ready to live a life without the fatigue and emotional pain?

Who will I be if my friends realize that I no longer am suffering?

Will I lose their friendship?

Will I lose their attention?

Will I lose this place where I'm living?

What's going to happen to me?

This is real scary.

This is terrifying.

I choose to let go of this fear.

When I am stuck in fear and doubt, it is impossible for me to think clearly.

As I let go of this fear of living with this condition . . .
. . . and then work with the fear of what will show up when I heal . . .
. . . I am ambivalent and wishy-washy about what I really want to manifest.

I'm going back and forth between independence and dependence.

That could be a root cause of my fatigue.

I really choose to be clear.

I choose to make clear, mature, and empowered decisions.

I choose to let go of the fuzzy thinking right now.

It's time for me to let go of the fear of moving forward.

Look at me, holding onto this fatigue and inertia, how silly . .
. . . when my mind and my spirit really want to go forward.

It's time for me to get out of this prison.

Anything could be better than where I am right now.

I choose to let go of the fear of moving forward.

I give myself permission to heal.

I give myself permission to let go of the fatigue.

I give myself permission to let go of the old beliefs that have held me back and made me sick.

It's time to let go of all of this old stuff right now.

I will be fine as I move forward in my life.

Moving forward is the best thing for me.

The universe really wants to support me in all ways to move forward.

Underneath the Arm:

I deserve to heal.

I deserve to be happy.

I deserve to have unlimited energy.

I deserve to have fun in my life.

I deserve to feel secure in all ways.

I deserve to allow myself to get beyond this fatigue and emotional pain.

I deserve to get beyond this fatigue and emotional pain.

I choose to let go of all of that old life that I've been living the past few years.

I choose to let go of this old life I've been living for the past lifetime.

Tap above the **Liver** on the right side – just below the rib cage.

My liver is overworked.

I love my liver.

My liver has done such a good job.

Right now, I choose to support my liver in its healing.

I choose to support my liver to let go of the rest of the toxins that are in my body.

I choose to send good energy to my liver.

I choose to allow my liver to gently let go of all the toxins and to stay healthy.

I choose to let go of all of my anger about being assaulted my whole life.

I choose to let go of all my anger that I carried in my DNA and past experiences.

It's really time to let go of all the anger that surrounds me now.

So I am happy to let go of this anger now.

I choose to let go of this anger now.

I choose to have a very healthy, happy liver.

Top of the Head point:

I am grateful to have learned many lessons in my life up till now.

I'm grateful that I can let go of all of the victimhood of my life now.

I am grateful that I know now that I deserve to heal.

I choose to heal.

God wants me to heal.

The universe is supporting me in all ways to heal right now.

And so it is."

Tapping Sequence 2 –

Gerry & Unworthiness

Even though Gerry reported to me needing help with her severe health issues, I discovered that she was really not emotionally open to receive help of any kind because on some level she believed that she did not deserve support and was not worthy of being healthy. This is the tapping sequence that opened her up to receive, and she later remarked that it was a real turning point in our work together.

You may follow along and tap on your own related issues.

> "Tapping at the **Karate Chop point:**
>
> Even though I have experienced some painful and terrifying events in my past . . .
>
> . . . I took on as a young person, even as an infant, that there was something wrong or bad with me.
>
> Rather than having the power at that young age to say that the negativity was coming from without, I took it in.
>
> Being helpless to defend myself, I took it in. I didn't know it wasn't me.
>
> Even though I misunderstood and I thought that I was bad . . .
> . . . instead of just receiving bad treatment from others I understand now.
>
> It's time for me to let go of the thoughts and beliefs of that young child, even though that will put me in the unknown and my first reaction is fear.
>
> Holding onto the negativity of other people is a painful place to be.
>
> My freedom will feel very, very good compared to how I feel

now.

Even though there is a place that I have never experienced
yet . . .
. . . I want to trust that letting go of this negativity has got
to be better.

I choose to trust that I can let go of this negativity that I
took on so, so many years ago.

I trust that when I'm connected to source and the universe
and that wonderful energy of the universe . . . that I am
safe.

Letting go of these old, stuck emotions of the past will allow
me to feel a clearer connection with source and the universe.

I don't feel very much of it. That's why it's my number one
priority.

My emotions and my ability to feel connected to a larger
purpose,
whole, divinity, have been constricted because of negativity.

I deserve to feel my source.

I deserve to feel my source. I don't know what that would
be. Wow. I'd like to know that.

For my whole life, that connection with the universe has been
blocked.

For my whole life, my sense of my connection with -- I think
it has been here because I'm still alive, but I'm not actively
able to feel it in ways that I want to.

I choose to clear that connection.

I choose to let go of this muddy energy around me.

I choose to let go of all the emotions related to my abuse.

I choose to let go of all of the old tendencies to beat up on myself and say that I deserved it.

I choose to be free of all of that old abusive energy.

I choose to be free of my belief that I deserved it."

At this point Gerry interjected: "I feel my resistance is up at ten right now. I'm aware of resistance. I wish it wasn't so."

I suggested that we continue, knowing that when the emotions are heightened the work and its results can be even more profound.

"Even though I feel like I deserved that abuse . . .
. . . and that I was not worthy of being treated nicely . . .
. . . and I was just a little kid that felt unloved . . .
. . . and that I really deserved to be punished and abused . . .
. . . now I really do understand and I deeply accept myself."

Just like many clients who have worthiness and self-love issues, Gerry was unable to repeat the classical EFT Set-up Statement: "Even though X is happening, I deeply and completely accept myself." She said that she could say "I deeply appreciate myself," but not the "completely" part. She also said she wasn't always able to say "I love myself," another statement often used in the EFT sequence.

It is beneficial to shift gears when issues or inner resistance shows up during a meridian tapping sequence because this often shows what the subconscious thrusts forward as the next and highest priority to clear. I follow that because each case is unique and the client's body-mind knows best. We continued.

"I'm doing the best I can do.

I've always done the best I can do.

I know this.

I accept this.

I give myself lots of credit for this.

Eyebrow point:

I felt like I deserved to be punished and abused.

I felt like I was unworthy of good treatment.

I must have been bad to deserve all that bad treatment.

I must have been unworthy or I would have received better treatment.

Outside Eye point:

I must have really been bad to deserve all that bad treatment.

What a horrible little girl I must have been to deserve that.

I don't know why else I would have been treated that way unless I deserved it and was bad.

Underneath the Eye:

They treated me like I was horrible and I just believed that I was.

They kept treating me badly and I just kept believing it, that I must be really bad.

I really don't deserve to love myself.

I don't deserve to be healthy.

I don't deserve to be happy.

I don't deserve to have abundance and love and income all around me.

I'm just a horrible person.

They treated me like I was and I believed it.

My whole life, I've believed that.

Under the Nose:

I must have been really bad when I was little to deserve that.

I must have done some bad things.

I don't even remember, but they must have been horrible.

I really must have deserved all that bad treatment.

When they stopped abusing me, I started abusing myself.

I went out in the world and attracted injuries and situations that would hurt me the way they used to.

That's all I thought I deserved.

Gee, I must have been really horrible.

Part of me thinks I still am horrible.

Part of me will not let go of this pain and the physical conditions right now.

I've gotten used to it and I don't deserve anymore. I don't deserve to be healthy.

This is what I deserve, to be in this body and this life situation as hard as it is.

I just believe it because of the way I started believing when I was an infant.

Chin point:

I must have done so many shameful things when I was little to deserve that.

I don't even remember what those shameful things could have been, but they must have been horrible.

I deserve to be abused and treated badly.

I'm still working out that old karma from those things I did.

They must have been really, really shameful.

Why else would I be living this life with this body with these problems?

I guess I just deserve to be living with these conditions the rest of my life.

All this is based on my first thoughts as an infant.

I've carried those old emotions for a really, really long time.

My belief system is based on those negative emotions.

Look at what I've created in my life.

Do I really want a life sentence of these conditions?

Do I really deserve that?

Is there anything that I could have done that was so horrible to deserve all this pain and suffering?

I was an infant. How could I have ever done anything so horrible?

Maybe I'm working out old karma in my DNA as well.

Maybe I'm even bringing in some old debt from a past life.

Maybe it's time to let go and say, "I've paid my dues."

I've suffered for many years.

I've lost almost everything.

I think and I believe that I have suffered enough.

That is why I am taking the time to do these exercises now.

I believe now that it's time to let go of the thinking and the old debts of an infant or a past life.

I think it's time to clear the slate and move forward.

It's time for me to connect with my true, authentic self.

It's time for me to feel the full, wonderful connection to the divine.

It's time for me to feel totally safe in all ways.

It's time for me to be open to learn new things and to set new beliefs . . .
. . . and to allow those beliefs to come through a different filter . . .
. . . to allow those beliefs to come to me freely without being put through a self-repulsion filter.

I choose to be open to let go of this old filter now.

I choose to be free to let go of these old emotions now.

I choose to reclaim my physical health now.

I choose to reclaim my personal power now.

I choose to allow myself to heal now.

I choose to allow myself to love myself now.

I choose to love myself now.

I love myself.

I deeply and completely accept myself.

I accept that no matter what I've done, I've always done the best I could do this life.

I trust that the energy of the universe is all-loving.

I trust that that energy is so much better than the stifled energy I have felt up till now.

I choose my freedom now.

It's time for me to let go of the old patterns and beliefs.

Let's go to the **Collarbone point:**

I was so afraid as a child.

I would do anything to keep from being treated badly.

I was afraid in many, many ways.

I'm still afraid of the unknown.

When I was a child, I never knew when something bad was going to happen.

I was always on alert.

I had to be on alert just to survive and protect myself.

Now, I don't have those same abusers around me.

I have a support team now.

I know people that love me and that support me.

I know that I have tools for transformation.

I know that I can gently and easily shift my beliefs.

I know that I have not been attacked recently.

I probably attracted those toxins to myself years ago because I was sending out a vibration to the universe to attract negativity.

I didn't like myself anyway, so why not tox out the body?

Those things have changed now.

I am ready to create a new life for myself.

I am ready to create a new body for myself.

I am ready for everything to change in positive ways.

I know that if I focus on the positives of what I want to manifest . . .
. . . and I really feel what it's going to feel like to be in that new life . . .
. . . then that will happen.

It is time to let go of the old blocks.

I choose to let go of the old blocks now.

They no longer serve to protect me.

I can protect myself in other ways.

I can let go of this fear.

I can let go of the fear of that infant and that small child . . .
. . . and I can move into my adult belief system.

I can recreate that belief system.

I really do deserve to be loved and to love myself.

I really do deserve to be healthy . . .
. . . and symptom-free.

This is what I choose.

Underneath the Arm point:

Even though before, I believed that I was unworthy of good things . . .
. . . I am changing that belief system now.

I am an adult with a whole different scenario around me now.

I choose to let go of the old emotions and beliefs of that young, young child.

Those beliefs are inappropriate for me as an adult now.

Those fears are inappropriate for me now as an adult.

I choose to let go of them now.

Top of the Head point:

I was abused as a child.

I was led to believe that I deserved it.

I felt like I was horrible.

I felt that I deserved to be punished.

I believed that I was a bad person.

I even used to hate myself.

I felt like I was really worthless.

Now I am choosing to change those beliefs.

I choose to let go of those old beliefs now.

I am a wonderful child of God.

The universe loves me.

The universe protects me.

I am safe.

I deserve to be healthy.

I deserve to be symptom-free.

I deserve to be free to love and to love myself.

I deserve all good things in life.

I am worthy of receiving them now.

And so it is."

Tapping Sequence 3 –

Gerry Disconnected from her God

This session was so potent for Gerry that it literally "knocked her out of her body". The first day after this session she slept for 9 hours... a lot for her. And for several days she woke up in a dazed "out-of-body" state... and, as she felt disconnected from her body, she didn't scratch.

It is amazing how many people have a fear that God doesn't love them or that God doesn't want them to be health, happy, secure, loved, etc. They "hide" from God. This sense of "disconnect" or unworthiness sometimes comes from church indoctrinations, sometimes from a personal sense of low personal regard, and sometimes from another "life" or experience with which the client relates and has felt abandoned, pushed away, or punished.

When such a core level disconnect is cleared there is always healing on some level. Some practitioners of NET/ Neuro Emotional Technique will first check the body for a "God issue" before doing anything else... just because this is so common and the re-connect can be so life-changing.

In this and other tapping sessions Gerry refers to God as "Source". This sequence focuses on her loss of faith and disconnection from her God. And, since Gerry's spirituality believes in reincarnation and past lives, she speaks to that as I direct her sequence.

We began by tapping on the **Karate Chop point:**

> "Even though I am afraid of the unknown . . .
> . . . and I'm comfortable with this feeling of resistance to connecting to Source.
> . . . and I'm used to it. It's familiar.
> . . . I'm familiar with this feeling of resistance . . .
> . . . and this disconnect from Source.
>
> It's an old pattern.

It just feels strange to be letting that go.

It feels scary to be letting it go. Who would I be?

I really do know that I choose to let go of this resistance.

I really do know that I choose to let go of this resistance. I want to find a way to feel safe letting go of it.

It's time for me to let go of it now.

Even though I'm afraid to let go of this resistance . . .
. . . and it feels scary because I don't know what's on the other side . . .
. . . and I don't know who I will be if I'm connected to Source . . .
. . . and I don't know who I will be if I am working with my full power . . .
. . . and I also don't know who I'll be if I let go of dependence . . .
. . . and I trust the process.

I trust my Highest Self...
. . . but I don't know if I do. That's the problem. I have confusion about if I'm connected, that's what brought disaster.

It's almost like I have a belief that being connected to Source brings disaster. That's what I would like to clear

I have this belief that being connected to Source brings disaster.

Even though I feel scared about getting connected to Source because I feel it means disaster will come about,
. . . I truly am willing and would like to release this fear and belief.

Even though I have an old belief that scares me . . .
. . . an old belief that if I connect with Source, disaster will follow . . .

. . . and I don't even know where that came from . . .
. . . and I do know where it came from, in a past life . . .
. . . but I don't know all the other past lives that may have had the same sequence . . .
. . . and I may not know all the past lives that have the same sequence . . .
. . . so I may not know the original occurrence of me taking on that vibration.

I sense this is one past life where that's what I carry with me.

This vibration that I did feel in that past life . . .
. . . I choose to let go of that old belief now.

I choose to let go of that fear of that vibration now.

I choose to change the way my belief system is accepting that.

I can let go of that fear. It was in a past life.

I can let go of that belief because it was based on false evidence appearing real.

I'm ready, willing and able to change my way of thinking right now.

I'm ready, willing and able to feel safe while being connected to source.

Eyebrow point:

I get angry thinking that I have been living with an old, false belief for so long.

I've been angry that I couldn't connect to Source out of fear.

It's time to let go of that anger.

It's time to let go of that fear.

It's time to let go of all anger that I had about my Higher Self.

It's time for me to let go of all anger that I projected toward God or towards Source.

End of the Eye:

I have felt resentment that after all the work I've done, I couldn't feel good about connecting to Source.

I feel resentment that after all the work I have done, I can't yet feel connected fully to Source.

I resent that I had a belief that it was dangerous to connect to Source.

I resent that I felt that God abandoned me.

I resent God that I thought he abandoned me.

I resented my Highest Self because that was disconnected.

It's time to clear all that old resentment.

I choose to let go of all that old feeling of resentment.

Under the Eye:

I have suffered for so long with this disconnection.

It's time for me to reclaim all the parts of me . . .
. . . and it's time for me to feel connected to my Highest Self . . .
. . . and in connecting to my Highest Self, I am connected to Source.

I choose to reconnect with my Higher Self.

I choose to feel really comfortable being connected to my

Higher Self.

I choose to feel really comfortable and proud to be really connected to my Higher Self.

I choose to let go of all emotions blocking me from this connection with my Higher Self.

I choose to let go of the fear that I felt that something bad might happen.

I see now that I can safely connect to Source and connect to my Higher Self.

I feel that I can safely connect to Source and to my Higher Self.

Tap **above the mouth and below the mouth**:

I choose to see beyond my mind and my ego self.

I can feel my inner self.

I know my intuitive self.

I know my Higher Self.

My Higher Self talks to my regularly.

I've always been connected to my Higher Self.

I felt like I had to disconnect from what I perceived as outside Source.

When every time I had a flashback of a past life or an insight, that was my connection to my Higher Self.

My Higher Self is part of Source.

All this time, I was still connected and I didn't know it.

My mind got in the way.

My mind was very busy and put up a set of beliefs.

The beliefs became very fearful to me.

I attracted some situations in my life that were very fearful to me.

I lived with a lot of fear. I was scared many times.

I felt disconnected because I was hiding and feeling this fear.

Actually, I was still connected but I couldn't feel that because I was surrounded by fear.

Collarbone point:

Even though I was very afraid in that past life . . .
. . . and even though I was very afraid this life as an infant and small child . . .
. . . it's time for me to let go of all that fear now.

I choose to let go of it now.

The fear has just been a burden to carry around.

The longer I held onto it, the more I attracted to myself.

I choose now to let it go for good.

I choose to be able to feel my real connection that's always been there.

I choose to know and to feel that I am totally safe being connected to Source.

Under the Arm:

I deserve to feel safe in my connection with Source.

I choose to feel excited and totally empowered in this connection with Source.

I've gotten rid of the wall now and I embrace that connection. I feel the flow coming into me.

I've released that wall and I embrace the flow and the feeling of that connection coming into me.

Top of Head:

I am grateful that I was always connected to Source.

I am grateful that God was always there watching over me.

I am grateful that I've always had freedom of choice.

I am grateful that I can let go of old, un-beneficial beliefs now.

I'm grateful that I have cleared the old fears that separated me from my feeling of empowerment.

And so it is."

Tapping Sequence 4 –

Gerry Loving Her Skin

During this session I suggested the following:

"If you are seeing psoriasis coming in new places like on your legs, because you can reach them, I suggest you do some experimenting. Test if you can use EFT in a topical way to keep the psoriasis from spreading, and to let go of the new breakouts. What I mean by that is, some practitioners of EFT and other related therapies will actually go to scar tissue and places where people have had operations and injuries or traumas to their body; they actually put one hand on the location of where that was and then they'll tap. They'll focus just on that specific thing.

I can create this little format. Let's make it comfortable. Sit in a chair and cross your leg. Touch the psoriasis where it appears. Put your hand over it. Lovingly say, 'I'm here to help you go way.' This is a manifestation of your body. You love your body. Doctors say, 'Oh, psoriasis is so horrible. You can't get rid of it.' Drugs won't get rid of it. Why? Because it's coming from inside. It's coming from your emotions. It's coming from your subconscious.

If you're sitting there with your hand over the psoriasis, you're talking to your body. Your subconscious is saying, 'I really love my body. I love my skin. I love the fact that my skin is the biggest organ. My skin can help me to let go of these toxins I've been carrying around. I'm breaking them loose on the inside, so my skin is a wonderful vehicle to let them go. I'm going to help my skin.'"

> "As you've got your one hand on the psoriasis, take your other hand and tap the **Karate Chop point**. Start your regular EFT protocol:
>
> Even though this psoriasis is showing up now on my legs, I know that it's my body's way of letting go of the toxins.
>
> Even though this is uncomfortable and I think it's kind of ugly, I know it's part of my healing process.

I am grateful that my body is healing itself through letting go of toxic things through my skin.

I choose to give my skin more energy to allow it to let the toxins go without creating psoriasis.

I choose to let my body let go of the toxins gently and easily without creating more problems on the skin.

It's my highest intention and I choose to do everything in my system that I can to help my skin be really healthy so it can continue to let go of all the toxins that I am letting go of on the inside.

I am committed to letting go of these toxins from the inside out.

My skin is the biggest, most wonderful, dynamic organ to let go of the residue and the nasty stuff that I am dislodging on the inside of my body.

I choose to support my skin in every way I can to let go of the toxins so that the skin can be made stronger and healthier as it lets the toxins go.

Even though the toxins are showing up as psoriasis on my skin, I deeply and completely love myself. I love my body. I appreciate this process of letting go of the toxins.

Just say that three times:

1- Even though my body is processing and letting go of the toxins, and the psoriasis seems to be showing up, I deeply and completely love myself and love my body and love my skin.

2- Even though my body is processing and letting go of the toxins, and the psoriasis seems to be showing up, I deeply and completely love myself and love my body and love my skin.

3- Even though my body is processing and letting go of the toxins, and the psoriasis seems to be showing up, I deeply and completely love myself and love my body and love my skin.

Eyebrow points:

I choose to make it as easy as possible for my body to let go of these toxins as I dislodge them emotionally from the inside out.

This psoriasis is evidence that my body is de-toxing.

This psoriasis can go away.

My body can support my skin to let go of these toxins.

I choose and I commit to helping my skin in every way possible to continue letting go of these toxins.

End of Eye points:

This skin is doing a wonderful job of letting go of these toxins.

This psoriasis is must evidence of the toxins going away.

I choose to let go of the psoriasis and create and support healthy skin so that the skin and tissue on my body can let go of all those nasty toxins I've been carrying for too long.

I'm going to do everything in my power to keep my skin healthy so it can let go of the toxins without the psoriasis.

Underneath the Eye, the same thing:

Even though I've got this condition on my skin, I know that my skin is de-toxing.

I know the toxins are leaving through my skin.

I know I'm continuing to de-tox.
I choose to let the toxins leave in many different ways.

I choose to support my skin to be as healthy as it can be so it can continue to let go of the toxins.

Other parts of my body can let go of the toxins, too.

If I keep drinking a lot of water, maybe my skin will have more resilience, more fluid in its tissue and will be able to release the toxins without the psoriasis.

Maybe it'll go through my bladder and other systems and I can let it go with urine.

Whatever it is, I'm committed to learn, if I don't already know, how to best support the detoxification of my body."

At the end of this session Gerry and I had a conversation where I asked her whenever she started to scratch to immediately grab her *Karate Chop point* and start tapping."

She said: "I do that and then I scratch as I'm hitting the *Karate Chop point*. I watch myself. I'm conscious of it. I know exactly what I'm doing. I'm scratching as I'm doing the *Karate point."*

So I asked: "Who's in control here? It sounds like you need to be in balance with yourself. See what feels good around the idea of the control, the habit, the discipline, the choice, the intention, the commitment. These are all your choices. When you're unconscious, you're unconscious. If you notice you're scratching, then you do have the power to do something about it. When you're conscious of that, you can make a change in that if you choose to do so. With that thought, I'm going to bid you a happy weekend."

The feedback from this session gave me a glimpse of good things to come, and also alerted me to the timing for her personal power session which came next.

Tapping Sequence 5 –

Gerry Reclaiming Power over Psoriasis

This is the final tapping sequence in Gerry's "Psoriasis Trilogy".

If you ask any doctor they will tell you that psoriasis seems to have a mind of its own, and cannot be controlled. When we go deeper than just the skin, by clearing old wounds and then coming back and filling in the gaps with personal power, the body will notice and results can be almost miraculous.

This is the final recording that helped to instill in Gerry her lost sense of personal power, and it was the final "icing on the cake" for her psoriasis journey. She had amazing results after this session, and we couldn't have done this "power session" without first clearing out her beliefs about unworthiness and self hatred.

Karate Chop point:

Even though my scratching hands are in charge of who I am . . .
. . . and while I'm tapping, they even take over and start to scratch . . .
. . . and I can acknowledge that I see them and they still scratch and don't stop . . .
. . . I feel like a victim to my hands.

My hands just take over and create chaos on my skin.

I just don't feel like I have any power over my hands.

There's part of me that wants to have psoriasis.

Part of me wants to make it worse.

Part of me wants to stay sick.

I still feel like a victim on some level.

At the same time, I deeply and completely accept myself.

I am complicated like every other human.

I just have some issues that I still need to clear.

I choose to clear those issues that are trying to take over control of my skin.

I choose to let go of all levels of victimhood.

I choose to allow my skin to heal.

It is time for me to let go of these hurtful and stressful old blockages.

I really deserve to have beautiful skin again.

I deserve to allow myself to love me.

I have the power to stop scratching.

I have a choice of using that power or not.

It is still my choice.

I can be a victim to the scratching or I can take control.

I can create triggers where, if I catch myself scratching, I can move my hands to do something else.

I can create triggers so when I notice my hand scratching, I can do something else.

I do have the power to take over the control over the healing of my psoriasis.

Just because genetically I inherited that opportunity to develop psoriasis from my mother . .
. . . and I have created stressful situations in my life . . .

. . . I still can let go of the stress and let go of the physical psoriasis.

It is my choice.

As long as I want to continue to have health issues, I will have them.

When I truly decide to get healthy and let go of all of the past and all of the self-contempt .
. . . then I can heal myself.
. . . then I will be healed.

I have all the power that I need right now.

I have all the power that I need right now.

And, I'm afraid of power. That's a problem.

That is an old belief.

From somewhere, maybe even a past life, I am afraid to misuse power.

From somewhere in a past life, I have been afraid to misuse power.

It was stuffed down so that I couldn't use power growing up.

It probably came from before that, either genetically or energetically.

I created a situation where I wasn't allowed to use my power growing up.

It was all based on my own fear of my power . . .
. . . and me misusing my power.

That could also be me misusing my energy . . .
. . . or me misusing energy exchange with others.

Something in my subconscious said that I was unable to use power in positive ways.

I believed that.

Now it's time to clear that belief.

I am aware of energy exchange and balance now.

I am aware that I can control my hands and stop the scratching.

I am aware that I can get out of victimhood.

I am aware that I can get out of victimhood and I thought I had.

I can change my perception about everything in my life.

I can easily take my power back and use it well.

I can take care of myself and that will be easy and fun.

If I've got some resistance about being self-sufficient . . .
. . . then I can let go of that, too.

I have the whole universe working for me right now.

All I have to do is let go of the blocks . . .
. . . and let go of the fear of moving forward into a wonderful, fulfilling life.

I have everything I need to create a perfect life for myself now.

I know that it is time for me to let go of the fragments that are left, that are still holding me back.

I choose to use my personal power to create my best life.

I choose for my personal power to be balanced and fun to

use.

I choose to be inspired as to the best ways to use my personal power.

I choose to start using this personal power to stop the scratching of the skin.

Eyebrow point:

I choose to let go of frustration and anger about the psoriasis.

I choose to let go of confusion about being a victim.

I choose to let go of all frustration around misusing personal power.

I choose to clear up the confusion I have about who's in charge here.

Ultimately, I am in charge.

Whatever I focus on, I can create.

I choose to be able to feel the subtle blockages as they come up and then clear them immediately.

I have this power.

I have these tools.

Whenever the feeling comes up of blockage or resistance . . . . . . it is my responsibility to clear it immediately.

Otherwise, I fall into victim mode.

Outside Eye point:

I have resented my skin since I got the psoriasis.

I've resented my mother's skin before I resented my own.

I resented my genes for allowing me to inherit that propensity to have psoriasis.

I've resented my body for a number of years.

My body is a wonderful model of deeper levels of blockages.

I realize that I have been clearing a lot of these old beliefs and blockages out.

They're gone now.

I'm going to a deeper layer.

I can feel resistances and clear them immediately.

I can let go of all resentment toward my body.

In fact, I am so grateful that my body is showing me things that I needed to clear.

My body is allowing me to really perform my soul contract.

The inner work is the ultimate work.

I might not have done it if the body hadn't shown me that it was blocked.

I'm grateful to my wonderful body.

I know that as I finish clearing out the blocks and the stresses . . .
. . . that my skin will clear up, too.

In the meantime, I choose to control my hands and control the scratching.

Under the Eye:

I have carried so much stress and negative charge in my body.

Sometimes my inner electro-magnetics are somewhat confused and in conflict with each other.

It's up to me to calm myself down . . .
. . . to look toward what I should be grateful for . . .
. . . to use calming techniques and gratitude . . .
. . . in addition to my tapping . . .
. . . so that I can continue to raise the vibration around my body . . .
. . . so it can feel more comfortable.

Oftentimes, the body is the last level to let go of the negativity.

It takes a while for cells to regenerate.

Maybe I've already let go of most of the stressors and energetic blockages . . .
. . . and it's just time for me to get out of the way, stop scratching and let the skin heal.

Sometimes the scratching is an unconscious habit.

Sometimes it is brought on when I feel energy shift in my body.

Sometimes it's just a nervous reaction that I've done for a long time.

I can control the scratching.

I choose to control the scratching.

I choose to be in control over my scratching fingers.

Tap **Above your lip and Below your lip** at the same time:

I've been so afraid of my personal power all of my life.

I believed that I would misuse personal power.

I believed that I'd be punished for using my power.

I believed I needed to be a victim in order to survive.

I got in trouble whenever I tried to use my personal power.

It's time to clear all of these old beliefs about power.

As a human being, I have personal power that was given to me when I was born.

It is my birthright to use my power.

It is my birthright to use my power.

I came to this planet to learn how to create a life.

I came to this planet to learn how to create a life and be in alignment with personal power.

When I use my personal power, I have the power to create the life of my dreams.

It's only old beliefs that have held me back this long.

As an abused baby, I believed it was dangerous for me to exert any power.

I was stifled and not allowed to use my power. It was unsafe.

Right now, many years later, I'm still living with the belief system of a preverbal infant.

Right now, 64 years later, I'm still living with the belief system of a preverbal infant.

It is hurting me every day.

It really needs to be dropped and let go of now.

I am safe now.

My survival depends on me using my personal power now.

My health and wellbeing depend on me taking my power back.

It is my birthright.

Even though I believed that I didn't have the power, I've always had it.

I just was blocked from using it.

I blocked myself from using my own personal power.

At my age now, I deserve to take that power back.

I choose to reclaim my power now.

It's way overdue.

It's perfect timing.

I'm ready now.

I can be in charge.

That doesn't mean that I have to control everything.

I can be clear about what I want and let the universe support me to receive it.

I need to believe and have trust now.

Even though I have doubted my power in the past . . .
. . . and I have felt like a victim . . .
. . . I choose to let go of that belief now.

I choose to change that belief into something more in alignment with who I am.

I have the power to create the life that I imagine.

I have the power to be clear about what I want in my life.

I can let the universe come up with the details and the how to's.

I'm getting really close to being able to do this in every aspect of my life.

Just looking back several months, my life has dramatically changed in so many ways.

I can see this evidence now.

I trust that things are changing.

They are improving in my life.

I'm feeling better every day.

I am seeing the beauty of life every day.

I am feeling these wonderful improvements in my life every day.

I choose to be clear . . .

I choose to be clear to let go of the blockages . . .
. . . so that I can flow forward knowing that I have the power . . .
. . . so that I can move forward knowing that I have the power . . .
. . . to be clear and focused on what I want.

The universe will provide it.

I know the universe has total abundance without any limitations.

There is plenty of money and love and health and opportunities and fun waiting for me.

I already see them coming into my life.

I'm experiencing some of it every day.

Collarbone point:

I've been afraid of getting to this point in my life.

I thought it would be really scary and dangerous.

Look at me, there's nothing to be scared of.

I'm sitting here on the telephone. I'm feeling comfortable.

My body is getting healthier. There's nothing to be afraid of.

Look at what I've manifested for myself just in this year, 2010.

My goodness, my life is different.

It's getting better every day.

Do I see any reason not to trust this process?

Only my subconscious has the old beliefs. As they come up and I feel anything that blocks me, I can let them go.

I'm in this place I've been afraid to be. The only things I notice are positive changes.

It's absolutely time to let go of all the old fears I had about moving into my personal power.

I really can create everything that I want in my life.

I'm surrounded by abundance every day.

If I don't feel it in my life, it's only because I'm blocking it.

I have the tools to clear the blocks.

I just need to do it.

I need to take that responsibility.

That's my daily job.

The payoffs are total abundance.

Under the Arm:

When I was born into a human body, my birthright included power.

That's power to create the life of my desire.

Old beliefs kept me from creating this wonderful life.

Old beliefs and old conditioning told me that I needed to be sick and a victim.

Now I realize that those were beliefs that were really un-beneficial to me.

Old beliefs and old conditioning told me that I needed to be sick and a victim.

They were based on old energetics in my DNA and in my infant perception.

I may have also had some bleed over from past lives and karma.

None of that really relates to where I am today.

All of those old energetics and beliefs can be let go of now.

I deserve to create my new life now.

My mother, where she is now, would bless me to do this.

She couldn't see beyond her own blocks when she was in her body.

Now, she has no blocks.

She can see how the beliefs that she taught me were incorrect.

She was doing the best she could do.

I choose to let go of all of the beliefs of my mother.

I choose to let go of all the beliefs of my mother and my father.

I choose to let go of all their doubts and criticisms.

I choose to let go of all their limitations on me.

I choose to just let go of the negative hold that they and their opinions have had on me being who I want to be.

I choose to let go of their negative opinions . . .
. . . on me being who I am meant to be.

My young child self believed I had to be approved of by my parents.

I realize that that is false and untrue.

I can let go of that old belief and realize that I am my own Divine Partner.

I have the responsibility of living up to my divine self-power.

It is my job to live up to the expectations of my Highest Self.

That is without judgment or criticism.

That is living up to my authentic self with pure love from myself.

Every day, if I find myself going to scratch, I will take my hand gently and say, "I love me too much to scratch and hurt myself."

I've been waiting my whole life to learn how to do this.

It's time to love me.

This is my number one job now.

It's true feeling, not just words.

Every day, I will take action to demonstrate my love for myself.

That is the ultimate job and the ultimate reward.

Top of the Head:

I have experienced so many aspects of life so far.

I really love that I have tools to continue to improve my life.

I choose to use my powers to show my love for myself.

I choose to stop scratching the skin.

I choose to allow myself to heal on all levels.

I choose to be inspired as to the appropriate actions to take.

I also choose to be inspired to know whenever I'm feeling like a victim . . .
. . . or whenever I'm putting out victim energy.

. . . or whenever I'm putting out victim energy, especially when it's unconscious.

I choose to be awake instead of unconscious.

I choose to be crystal clear about how I feel.

I choose to tap away any feeling that feels less than optimal.

I choose to do this whenever a negative feeling arises.

I have the power and the ability to do this.

I can choose to skip it or do it. That is still my choice.

I know I've got the power to heal myself.

And so it is."

Gerry used this script on her own numerous times in the following days and weeks and found that she went longer without itching than she had for the entirety of the condition – over 13 years.

Tapping Sequence 6 –

Gerry's Dreaded Tooth Extraction

Some physicians believe that MCS is psychological, based on the body's reaction to a fear perception that any smell or unknown substance is poisonous and will cause a negative physical reaction.

This sequence is an example of how via meridian tapping one's perception of a future event can be shifted so that the end occurrence has no trauma or stress.

Months after this Dental Extraction session, Gerry realized that she dreaded a long drive to visit her daughter, and she expected the worst. After re-framing her expectations, as we did in the following dental tooth extraction tapping sequence, this is what she said:

> "GREAT use of tapping. I was very apprehensive of driving 3.5 to 4 hours (each way) to my daughter's and also driving on a 4-lane very busy highway part of the way (I hadn't done that in 14 years). My charge was at a 10+ and by spending over an hour at a time with the feeling state (of my fears) I got it to ZERO! And stayed that way all day in terms of driving!"

It turns out that she had to drive back on that same day, so this tool was a true life-saver for somebody who had not exerted in such a way for many years.

Here is the Dental Extraction Tapping Sequence from which Gerry later created her Dreaded Drive experience. The general "taking charge" energy that you can "tap in" with this sequence can be applied to any "dreaded" activity or upcoming event.

Start with tapping the **Karate Chop:**

Even though I've always had the power to be in the driver's seat and to be consciously driving my life . . .
. . . when I was a little girl, my mom . . .
. . . took away that feeling of power.

I never knew that I had that power.

I was afraid of exerting my power.

I was afraid of exerting my power because it looked like her rage.

It also might encourage her rage against me.

It also probably would have encouraged her rage against me. That was terrifying.

Now I realize and I love myself for it . . .
. . . that I've always had this power.

Now I am living a safe life as an adult.

I can put my hands on the steering wheel and consciously be in charge of my life.

I've always had this power and I never knew I could do it.

I've always had the power and I was afraid to exert my power.

This is based on the beliefs of a little, tiny girl.

What was valid for me when I was a little girl . . .
. . . is now old information.

I'm an adult and I am in charge.

It is safe for me to be in charge of my life.

I choose to be in charge of my life now.

Even though I have been feeling like a victim of my life circumstances for so long . . .
. . . and this probably came because I was abused as a child
. . .

. . . and I was never allowed to exert my power over my life . . .

. . . so I believed that that power was permanently taken away from me.

Now I know that I've always had the power.

It's time for me to use it consciously.

I'm excited and I feel safe to use it consciously now.

Eyebrow point:

It makes me frustrated to think I wasted so much of my life not using my power.

I can let go of this frustration and pick up that power now.

I can be consciously in charge and be totally safe doing it.

I can let go of the old belief that dental work has to be traumatic.

I had some past experiences where I was a victim of that.

I didn't enjoy the experiences. They were bad.

The experiences were horrible.

Now, I can choose my experiences.

I can consciously imagine that it's going to feel really comfortable and it's going to be an easy procedure for me.

I'll be pain free afterwards and I'll heal very quickly.

I can control this with my mind.

I've always had this power and I didn't know it.

Outside Eye point:

I resent that it's taken me this long to know that I had all this power.

My goodness, how much time I've wasted in my life.

Now I see my life getting better and better and I am going to be conscious about continuing this process.

I know now that I have let go of so many pieces of blockage in my filter.

I see things appearing in my life and changing in my life every day now.

It feels so good.

I'm so excited.

Life gets better every day.

I can consciously keep this happening.

I choose to do that.

Under the Eye:

It disgusts me to think that I had all this power the whole time . . .
. . . and I didn't even know it.

Now I know it's safe for me to use my power.

I can be conscious about how to use it in a very balanced way.

I'm going to consciously be in charge of creating my life from the inside out.

I know that I can hold the feeling and change my vibration.

I choose to do this for the rest of my life to create the life of my dreams.

Under the Nose:

I gave away a lot of my personal power as a child.

I gave away all of my personal power as a child.

I'm just starting to reclaim it now.

It's time for me to be back in charge of my life.

I can do this in a gentle, vibrational way.

It will feel really safe and comfortable to me.

It's my inner work of being conscious.

People on the outside will feel it and it will feel very good to them . . .
. . . because it will be just the raising of my vibration.

I'll be able to do this on my own.

I am now consciously taking charge of my personal power.

It feels good.

Chin point:

Wow! I really signed on for a difficult contract when I was born.

I'm glad the hard work is behind me.

Now I see the light.

Now I know that I've had this power all along.

All I have to do now is consciously focus and create.

I'm not even tempted to go out and try to move mountains.

My weakened body couldn't move mountains anyway.

I have a perfect opportunity to see the power of working from the inside out.

I have the perfect opportunity . . .
. . . of experiencing working from the inside out . . .
. . . and feeling how life can totally change just by me feeling a different vibration.

That is where my power is.

That is where I can put my focus now.

Wow! This is exciting.

Collarbone point:

I have lived with lots of fear in my life.

I can let go of that because it was put there as an infant.

Even more recent fears having to do with dentists and doctors, I can let go of these, too.

Even though I have been afraid to have this dental procedure done . . .
. . . I can feel it happening very painlessly and easily.

Anytime fear and doubt come up during the procedure, I can tap my *Karate Chop*.

I know that I can let go of all the remnants of the old fear and replace that with trust.

My mind can totally turn off any pain and it can heal the space immediately if I focus.

I have that power.

I choose to let go of all old fears that I've been carrying around.

I choose to let go of all old fears about dental work that I've been carrying around.

I can be in charge of how I feel.

I have that choice and that power.

Under the Arm:

I deserve to use this power that I've always had.

I am so excited to be reminded that I have that ability.

I am going to accept the responsibility of consciously using my power . . .
. . . because it's a wonderful privilege.

It was a privilege and a gift given to me when I was born.

I am so grateful for now knowing that I have this gift of power.

I feel like being conscious and in charge of my life is a wonderful blessing.

I am grateful for it.

Top of Head:

I am grateful that I finally am realizing what I can do to create my own life.

I have struggled a long time to finally be able to realize this.

I am very grateful for the privilege of consciously taking my power and using it.

And so it is."

Gerry reported the following in her Post-Coaching feedback:

"As I said in my email, I appreciated our session because Friday I had a tooth extraction. I did have one three years ago. It went okay. I did have some reservation. As a result of our session, I went and was able to go there, be there in the chair. Even as the procedure was being done, I had a felt sense of a positive outcome and that I could literally notice how I felt a little afraid. It wasn't just like a thought, like an affirmation in my mind, but I just let myself feel.

I had two images that I would just go between. One was that at the end of the day, I would feel well enough that I could go up to my friend's house and see her two kids. The other one, I actually imaged myself writing a thank you note to the dentist. I had really intended to listen to our session again on my iPod. For some reason, I downloaded it, but it didn't play. I had listened again to it twice that night. It was still in my mind. Even though I didn't actually get to listen as I was in the chair, I had the thoughta pretty fresh with me.

This dentist is someone I continue to have confidence in. I've only seen him three times. Even though I was doing my own inner work, after he gave me the anesthetic, he touched the tooth a little and then said, "I'd just like to let the ligaments settle and relax. While they're relaxing, I invite you to take some time to say goodbye to your tooth and to thank it for all the good work it has done.

About ten minutes later, he came back and was literally able to just pull out the tooth effortlessly."

I believe this goes to show the power of mind over body, and the influence of changing the vibration of one's perception so that others react to it.

Tapping Sequence 7 -

Veronica

Veronica's life had been full of stress to such an extent that she lived in a state of perpetual hyper vigilance. Here is the tapping sequence that we used to clear a variety of stressful memories, issues, and old patterns that had caused her diagnosis of Hashimoto's Thyroiditis Disease.

Starting at the **Karate Chop Point**, I'm going to lead you just as I led Veronica in this session. What I'd like you to do is to make the statements, changing the words to best relate to your situation. You can say more or use words that are more in your own vocabulary. I also added for Veronica, that when she did tapping for herself, to do it in Italian, her native language, to find it more beneficial. We hold our native language in a different part of the brain than we hold second and third languages. She could tap and speak in English, too, but I think usually one gets more emotional release from his or her dominant language, and in Veronica's case much of her trauma occurred while growing up speaking Italian in Italy.

> "Even though I know that I was really stressed out by my dad
> . . . I deeply and completely accept myself.
>
> Even though he was really scary most of the time . . .
> . . . I know I was a good girl.
>
> I did the best I could do all the time.
>
> I know that even though he was very irrational sometimes
> . . . and I never knew what to expect from him . . .
> . . . I was always trying to be ready for the unexpected.
>
> Now my life is different.
>
> Now I can relax more.

It's appropriate for me to relax more.

It's safe for me to relax now.

It's safe for me to let go of this stress and being on guard.

It is good for my health for me to relax more.

I'm safe from my father now.

I know my husband and my son love me.

I have many loving friends.

I'm safe away from my father.

He cannot hurt me anymore.

Even though I know that my brain is still trying to protect me from my father . . .
. . . I deeply and completely accept myself.

I choose to get well.

I choose to support my body to rebalance.

It's safe for my body to be healthy now.

I'm living a good life now.

I'm safe in my new life.

I'm surrounded by love in my new life.

It's fun living where I live.

I choose to have my health in my new life.

I choose to help myself get well.

I know I can do this."

Let's go to the **Eyebrow Points**. That's right on the beginning of the hair of the eyebrows above the nose. Tap on each side with one finger on each side. Scan your body for any symptoms or sensations of stuck energy or emotion.

I asked Veronica to think about all the confusion she had about why she got sick with all the different aspects of this illness.

> "Why is my body beating up on itself? Why is it trying to destroy its own thyroid? What is it I really would like to tell my father?" I asked her to think about what she'd really like to tell him. "If you went back and watched him and the way he acted, and you were watching him treat you badly as a little child, what would you as an adult tell him now? You're a mother. You can talk to him as a father. What would you tell him now?"

Veronica replied in her own words:

> "I would never do that to my child. Why would you do that?
>
> You hurt me a lot. It was quite scary growing up with you. Whatever I did was never good enough. Even if I tried, my best was never good enough anyway.
>
> Part of me understands because you did what you did probably because of your parents doing that to you. Still, it's hard to accept in any way what you did."

When I asked Veronica to think back to the worst memory of her childhood with her father, on a scale of 0 being feeling no charge to 10 being a lot of charge, she said she felt a 6 on the particularly horrible memory she brought up.

I guided her to go to the **Ends of the Eyes** *points* to focus on how she felt as she focused on that memory... especially the worst part of that memory.

> "Just breathe it out. Let it go. That was a long time ago. It's making you sick to hold onto it anymore. It's

unbeneficial to hold onto this memory. Just let it go.
Breathe it out. Let it go.

Now go to the point **Under the Eye**.

"Breathe in a big breath of pure love. Feel it coming into
your body and filling you up with pure love. Just breathe it
out. Take one more big breath of pure love. Breathe it out.
Now I want you to go back to that really bad memory and
breathe in another big breath of pure love and send it to this
memory. Send it to yourself first. You really deserved
better treatment. You deserved to be loved by your parents
and treated well. And your father deserved to be loved by
his parents and treated well. You both needed that love.
Just breathe it out. Breathe in another big breath of pure
love. Send it to both you and your father and your siblings,
anyone else who was there. Breathe out the old hurt, the
pain that all of you suffered. Breathe it out. Take in another
big breath of pure love. Feel it coming into you and your
father and your siblings and your mother. Now breathe out
the hurt that all of you were suffering, the pain that all of
you were suffering, the confusion that all of you were
suffering, the impatience, the frustration. Just let it all go.
It was just so hurtful. All of you suffered."

Next go to the points **Above and Below the Mouth**.

"Think about the statement: 'My best never seemed good
enough for you.' I want you to think back to the things that
you really tried to do well, and you knew that you did them
well, but you never got any praise. You didn't get a pat on
the back. You didn't get any positive reinforcement. You
didn't know even doing something good might have triggered
your father to get angry. Even when you were trying to be
helpful or trying to help him or to be a good girl, sometimes
you still got beaten. It's time to clear that now and forever.
Think about a memory that holds a lot of fear because you
had no idea that in doing something good you were going to
get punished, or he was going to yell at you or tell you it was
bad, or you didn't do it well enough. You knew that you put
effort into what you were doing. Just breathe out the hurt.

While you're tapping there with one hand, I want you to put the **other hand right at your solar plexus**, which is right above your navel and below your ribcage, right in that central diaphragm area of your body. That's your power center, your **third chakra**. Living with people like your father, who did not see the good in you, who could not see the good in you, who could not recognize when you did a good job – maybe he never told you he loved you. Maybe he never told you that you did a good job on anything because he couldn't. At the same time, that kind of took your power away. You felt like you had no power. 'If my daddy doesn't tell me good things, I must have something wrong with me. I must not be worthy of love. I must not be worthy of praise. Maybe I did do something wrong. Maybe I shouldn't have been born anyway. My mother didn't even want me. Why should I even be here? Why not kill myself from the inside out?' It's all connected. Just breathe that out. It's okay.

I know I did the best I could do in every moment.

I know I tried to be a good girl.

I was a good girl.

Even though I didn't feel like my parents really wanted to have kids . . .
. . . I am here and I am a good person.

As a mother, I let my son know how much I love him all the time.

I know what good parents are supposed to be like.

Unfortunately, my parents just didn't know.

They were probably doing the best they could do.

They still hurt me.

Both of them hurt me.

They never gave me the love that I deserve.

Now I choose to let myself know how much I love myself.

From now on, when I go and see myself in the mirror, the first thing I'm going to do is tell myself: 'I love you.'

I'm just going to tap in that energy because it's true. 'I love myself.'

I have created a new life filled with love.

I am using these tools to let go of all the unworthiness that I grew up with.

Let's move down to the **Collarbone Point**, which is at the base of the neck, right under the collarbones on both sides, at the top of the ribcage. Just tap there.

When I checked in with Veronica about any residual charge on that worst memory with her dad she reported that she felt around 2 out of 10.

I asked her to focus on the statement: "My best was never good enough for you." She had no charge on that.

She also had no charge left on the thought: "I was never good enough for dad."

When we brought up the next statement she still had the charge of 7 to 8 out of 10: "Mother, I know that you never really wanted me."

This happens with any surprise birth, any first child who was an early pregnancy. In Veronica's case, her dad wanted to have children and her mother really didn't. She made it real clear to Veronica and her sister that she really didn't want children. That hurts a lot.

I reminded Veronica to keep tapping at her **Collarbone** area... and you should, too. So many people with autoimmune have low self-worth because of something like this. It's very normal.

> "Just think about your mom. When you found out you were pregnant with your son, you were really surprised, too. You were probably happy, but you were surprised.
>
> In the case of your mother, she may not have even been surprised, but she was not happy. She couldn't get any support for keeping it from happening, or from how she felt because your father wanted to have children. He was not a great dad, but something in him said he was supposed to be a father.
>
> Think about your mom as you tap. Maybe she wasn't really appreciated by her parents.
>
> She had a bad childhood. Maybe she was very afraid that she couldn't be a good mother because she didn't have a good mother. Just breathe that out. You know how it is to be a mother. You know it's not an easy thing. It's a fulltime job. It takes your body, your mind, and your spirit to be a good mother. It's a very big commitment and your mother wasn't ready to make it, maybe never would have wanted to make it. Maybe later she grew to love you. Maybe later she really appreciated having daughters.
>
> ...but not toward the beginning. Let's go back to that statement: 'I didn't even want you and your sister.'"

Veronica reported that the statement felt a bit better but still held a 4 or 5 out of 10.

> "Great. Now go back to a memory with your mother where you just didn't feel like you were loved. You felt like she didn't want you and then she didn't love you. 'I feel like I don't even have a mother.' Go back to that memory with your mother where you just really felt like she didn't love you.

Let's say a few things to your mother here. What we're going to do is to tap on the **Under the Arm Points** while we talk to your mom.

Even though you didn't seem like you loved me . . .
. . . I loved you.

Even though it was difficult for you to have children . . .
. . . and sometimes I understand because I'm a mother . . .
. . . I deeply and completely love myself.

Even though you didn't have the capacity to love me . . .
. . . I do have that capacity to love me.

I also have the capacity to be a loving mother to my son.

Even though I did not learn good mothering skills from you
. . . I am a naturally good mother.

I appreciate that about me.

I love who I am.

Even though you couldn't love me when I was growing up . .
. . . I turned out to be a wonderful person.

I know how to give love and receive love.

I have created a beautiful life now.

I deserve to be healthy.

I have been sick long enough.

It's safe for me to be healthy.

It's appropriate for me to be healthy.

My son and my husband want me to be healthy.

I choose to be healthy so I can be a strong mother and wife.

I choose to be healthy so that I can be happy and have fun.

It's my God-given right to be healthy in this body.

I choose to reclaim my health now.

I choose to get back in balance with health.

I choose to speak my truth.

That is my God-given right also."

Let's go down to the **Side of the Legs**, one of several large intestine points. Tap on the outside of the legs. It might feel a little sensitive to you. It's not only a good place to tap for the large intestine, but it's a neurolymphatic reflex point that relates to your large intestine. If you're having trouble digesting or you're constipated, the sides of your legs are a wonderful place for you to rub. Especially if you feel a sensitive place, just rub that sensitivity out until it's no longer sensitive. You'll find it will either help you eliminate or it will just make you feel better. Now we're just tapping there.

"Even though I grew up in a household with a lot of stress and tension . . .
. . . I deeply and completely accept myself.

Look how wonderfully I turned out.

I'm really a success story looking at where I came from.

Even though I didn't receive the love that I felt I deserved . .
. . . I feel lots of love in my life now.

Even though I suffered and was traumatized when I was growing up . . .
. . . I can live a peaceful, balanced, happy life now.

I know that my family and friends love me.

I feel safe."

Now go to the **Top of the Head.** Bring in a feeling of gratitude. Breathe in a big breath of gratitude and feel just how grateful you are for the wonderful life you're living now.

> "You've escaped. You have love all around you. You're living a totally different life than you used to live.
>
> Let's go back and focus on that stressful job that you were in that pushed you over the edge. Let's clear that. Just breathe it out. That's all in the past. That was just a trigger even though it was really hard on you and not fun. You didn't like the place and you didn't like the people. You had to stay there. It was like living with your family. You didn't feel any love. There was a lot of stress in your family. You couldn't leave home because you were just a little girl. You were trapped in both places. We're letting go of that pattern forever. I want you to feel the gratitude that now your husband has a job, now you're in a different location, and you're not in that old job and not in that old family. Just feel gratitude for this new life that you're living and how wonderful it is."

Obviously you weren't living Veronica's story, but we're all connected in the human experience. A lot of what Veronica went through we all have suffered. We've each got our own version of Veronica's story. By tapping along with her story we can support ourselves to clear any related aspect in ourselves so that we don't have to suffer from that anymore.

When Veronica and I went back to her old issue that she knew her mother didn't want to have kids, with specific focus on the statement where her mother had actually said: 'I don't want you or your sister.' Veronica said she no longer felt any emotional charge. She also reported that she felt no charge regarding feeling unloved by her mother.

We ended with Veronica feeling lighter - with a large smile on her face.

Tapping Sequence 8 –

Helen

I asked Helen to tap on the **Heart Center** to engage the subconscious and energy system as we go over her history:

"Your mom is not around. She's an absent parent. Many of us have had absent parents. Sometimes it's the father; sometimes it's the mother. For whatever reason, whether they love us greatly or not, they're working or they're somewhere else, or we just think they're not loving us or not around even though maybe they just go to work and come home at night and come home at night tired and don't have time for children. In your case, she really wasn't there. She traveled for months at a time. You had that predisposition. You moved as a child to a different climate, which can have a physical impact.

So you had an absent mom and you really missed her. Whether it was really conscious all the time or subconscious, you had the missing mother. Then you moved and your body was hit with this new climate, new environment.

I miss my mom.

Where is she?

Now I'm with my dad fulltime.

He's different than he used to be when Mom was around.'

It could have just been any number of reasons why you had asthma. You were with a person who was very strict. And he had a temper. And he was mean to you sometimes.

We all have skeletons in our closet. Some people do their best but their personality is just not a good daddy personality, or they get frustrated, or they just can't handle it. For whatever reason, he was like a bomb ready to go off sometimes.

Everybody is always being the best that they can be in every moment. He was trying his best but his best was all you got. Whether that was good or bad, it wasn't easy. Let's focus on that. We're kind of thinking it through and then we're going to do some specific EFT for this. Here you were with a man who has temper outbursts, is definitely psychologically abusive, and sometimes even physically abusive. He just kind of blows his top and you're the nearest thing around.

He's just doing his thing, trying to be the best person he can be, but you're the little one. You're receiving this and not understanding it and missing your mommy. He's trying to control you.

The controlling energy is what you feel in your body. You're not only missing your mom, but you've got your dad trying to control you and it's tough.

He's making my life miserable and I don't really know when he's going to blow up at me.

It's hard keeping him happy.

Just when you thought you had your freedom - you didn't. You went to school one place and then your parents both said you had to come back and go back to school in Dad's country.

That was quite a devastating shock for my system.

That was very upsetting.

It all just caved in. Nothing went to plan basically.

They brought me home and said I'm going to go to school here.

That is when I really started having the skin problems.

I'm just going through this talking as you're tapping on the **Heart Center** to allow your subconscious to hear the rationale, to know that we are on your side. We're seeing why your wonderful subconscious, your wonderful part of yourself that really runs the show was trying to give you indicators a long time ago and was trying to rebalance and get well and push out the toxins. In this case the toxins were emotional. Then they became climate-based toxins with the climate changes during your moves. Then they became toxins with the metal poisoning. You've had all kinds of things coming into your life, and all of them affected the same energy circuits that needed some attention. That's what we're going to focus on today, the loss of your mom because of travel, loss of your freedom because you were around very dominating and controlling energy coming from your father, sometimes your mother, circumstances, university, even maybe some of the people at that wedding that you mentioned.

As a child I felt unsafe.

I felt hopeless and depressed.

I was helpless and they controlled me.

I think this is just the way it's always going to be.

Part of me is ready to give up.

Mom is always going to be away for a long time and then come back.

Mom is never going to be constantly at home with me.

I am very lucky now, however, because my mom lends me her frequent flier miles when I need to travel to see relatives.

My little inner child doesn't really delight in these benefits because she is still hurting."

Let's go to the **Karate Chop Point** now, which is the side of the hand.

> "Even though I have missed my mother since almost the day I was born . . . I know that she is still available to me now.
>
> On the day I was born, she looked at me and said: 'I've got to go back to work.'
>
> Just feel that energy and breathe it out as you tap.
>
> Even though I have felt this way since I was a little girl . . . I choose to let go of the pain.
>
> Just feel that. Feel how it felt. Your mom didn't consciously abandon you because she's still very much in your life, but she had to go back to work. That's where she spent most of the time you've been on the planet. She worked all the time. You know how that feels. It's just that hole in your heart.
>
> Even though I have felt this, I choose now to let this go.
>
> It is appropriate for me to let this pain go.
>
> It's time for me to let go of 23 years of that pain.
>
> Part of me doesn't want to let it go.
>
> Even though part of me doesn't want to let go of that feeling . . .
> . . . I know that it doesn't help me.
>
> It's unbeneficial to me.
>
> It's unbeneficial to my mother.
>
> It's unbeneficial to my father.
>
> It has no effect on my mother or my father.
>
> It's not really punishing them.

Even though I have felt all this pain and grief and even anger, it's not affecting them.

It's affecting me and my health.

It's time for me to let it go.

I choose to let it go.

I don't want to let go of the pain because it keeps them away. If they come close, maybe I'll get hurt.

Wait a minute. If they come and take away my freedom, or my father comes and brings up some really bad stuff. . .
. . . I don't need this. I might get hurt.

Even though part of me won't let this pain go because it thinks it's keeping them away so I don't need to feel the pain of loss when they leave,. . .
. . . I choose to understand fully that actually keeping this skin pain is keeping the pain of loss with it.

This stuckness is keeping me sick.

It's hurting my body.

These old emotions are hurting my body, and hurting my skin now.

But I still feel it's unsafe.

Even though I feel it's unsafe . . .
. . . I choose to let go of that feeling.

I choose to allow myself to be a 23-year-old adult that knows how to live without being oppressed by my parents.

I'm still young but I'm a young adult now.

I do love my parents.

Every time they leave, it hurts.

It's happened so many times in the past.

I just hate going through that every time.

There are times when I just really want to go with my mother.

Maybe sometime in the near future I will be able to create a way that I can go with her.

I could really get to know her and know if we could be friends.

Maybe see if she and I really do have anything in common or not as adults.

Even though it hurt horribly when I was a little girl and my mom would leave . . .
. . . and it still hurts now that I'm 23 when she leaves . . .
. . . I have a life now.

I have my own friends.

I have things that I do regularly in my life.

I can have an airline ticket anytime I need to go see her if it's an emergency.

I can email her or Skype her every day if I feel like it.

I have that freedom.

As a little girl I never had that.

Now my dad is not in my life fulltime like he used to be.

I have a lot less to be afraid of than ever before in my life.

That feels good.

Even though it still hurts when my mother leaves . . .
. . . I choose to let go of that excruciating pain.

I know that she is out earning money and having a life.

I'll be earning money and having a life soon, too.

She's a wonderful model if it's to be a career woman.

I also know how I would want to treat my child because I
know what I have missed.

I've got the best of both worlds going for me as an adult.

Even though it has hurt every time she's left me in the past .
. .
. . . from now on, I choose to feel less pain when she leaves.

I also choose to be proactive and reach out to her whenever
I want to talk to her.

I could be the one that initiates a friendship.

Instead of just being a needy little girl, I can be an adult and
create a relationship with my mother as two adults.

Even though when I was a child it really, really hurt . . .
. . . I choose to fill that heart with wonderful healing energy.

I choose to feel the love because it must have been hard for
my mother to leave all those times, too.

If I don't let them in, I won't feel the good stuff either."

Let's go to the **Eyebrow Points**.

"Go back to the times when you were alone with your dad.
He didn't really want to be a fulltime dad. Whether he really
wanted your mom around or not, he didn't have her either.

She was off. He was stuck with being an only parent.

Feel the confusion. You were a little girl and you're picking up on the fact that your mom has to leave and she goes away, so your own pain, but your dad's upset, too. He misses her. He wants her around. Now he has this little bundle of joy who's you, but he doesn't know how to be an only parent. He doesn't know what to do with this little baby and his wife is gone. He didn't know when he got married that she was going to be gone all the time either, let alone that he was going to have to raise you. You're picking up on his energy and your energy and your mom's energy. And, if they were fighting, you were picking up on that energy too. He was just trying to control his environment and you were part of that environment. Yes, he was controlling you.

I'm confused. I'm frustrated.

My dad is really impatient. He's getting really pissed off at mom, at the situation, at me.

He's got to change a diaper. He's got to feed me. He's got to do all this stuff about schedule. 'Where's my wife? She's off gallivanting across the world.'

The money probably wasn't a problem, but there you are and you're a big responsibility. If he lost his temper, maybe he felt bad about it later, but you didn't know that. Maybe he was trying to be a good dad but he didn't know how to be an only dad. Maybe he was frustrated about getting married and having a baby right away and his wife being gone. Then you're confused. He's a messed-up guy. He doesn't know what's going on. Here you're just a victim. You miss your mommy. You're crying for your mommy. Daddy's in a bad mood. He's grumpy because he's missing her, too, so he takes out his grumpiness and anger on you. He doesn't understand. You didn't do anything wrong.

It wasn't my fault I was born.

It's okay to be confused.

It's okay to be frustrated when you're a little one.

Now let's get rid of this. It just clutters your mind. You've got the rest of your life to live. Just breathe out all this frustration that you were picking up from everybody."

Let's go to the **End of Eye**.

"I want you to feel the anger and resentment that your parents probably felt. Your dad might have resented that your mom got pregnant with you. She might have resented that she got pregnant because of your dad. Then they both might have resented the situation that their freedom was gone because they had a child. She resented having to even consider quitting her job. Then he resented it because she was traveling and he was at home. You were picking up all this resentment, even if it wasn't yours. That could blow your head off right there.

Now tap into your own resentment. You want to be free. They wanted to be free, too. You inherited that in your DNA. You're all suffering from the same: 'I resent that there are other people and situations that are keeping me from living the life I really want to live.' Just breathe that out. That's a heavy emotion to be carrying. It's unbeneficial to you. It's unbeneficial to them. Nobody wins when you're just all feeling resentful. Just breathe it out. It's okay. It's in the past. You don't have to go back there anymore. It's over. It's time now.

I choose to let this go now.

I've lived with it for 23 years and I can stop it now.

Breathe it out."

Let's go **Under the Eye**.

"Now go back to feeling all the different feelings your mother felt: 'Uh-oh, I'm pregnant. Uh-oh, this guy and I are making a baby together. What are we going to do now?' All those feelings. And your dad, too, all the feelings he must have had. 'You're pregnant? Oh, my goodness!' You're picking up every single emotion that's around your mother while you're in her body. Let go of those things. 'We've got to get married. We've got to bring this baby up. I'm not quitting my job. I'm going to travel.' All the frustrations, all the confusions, all the strategizing, all the decision making. You, on some level, felt responsible for their unhappiness. You took away their freedom. Part of you feels guilty for that.

Tap that away.

You guys were adults. You didn't have to do it. Here I am, the best thing that ever happened to either one of you!

Even though part of me feels bad that I cramped your style . . .

. . . I choose to let go of that guilt.

It's just a weight that is unnecessary for me to carry for the rest of my life.

I choose freedom for all three of us."

Let's go to the points **Above and Below the Mouth**.

"I want you to feel any sense of that guilt or shame. There might have been times when you were a little girl and children's parents came to school or their mommies were there and your mommy was traveling. It's hard for a little one to explain that. Any sense of the dynamics that you were in or the feeling of: 'I'm guilty for cramping my mother's life or holding my parents captive.' Just breathe that out. Guilt is a heavy, heavy feeling. It is unbeneficial to everybody, without any benefits. Nobody benefits from guilt. Just breathe it out."

Let's go down to the **Collarbone Point** again, and tap there until you feel a shift on the following:

"I'm unsafe.

I'm feeling unsafe in society.

I don't know enough to feel safe."

Let's go to the spleen points, **Under the Arm**. Just tap there and repeat:

"I love myself.

Even though I have problems loving myself . . .
. . . I choose to let that go now.

Even though I have an old pattern of feeling guilty about my situation with my parents . . .
. . . it's okay and I am definitely lovable.

Even though my mother left me regularly, she still loves me.

She loves me as much as she is able to.

I believe this.

I love myself.

I'm a survivor.

I've always done the best I could do in every moment.

I know I have a bright future ahead of me.

I've got so much talent.

I've got potential.

I am a unique being with my own unique talents.

These will be unfolding the rest of my life.

I'm getting rid of this stuff that's holding me back from

seeing the abundance all around me.

When it's gone, my life is shifting for the better.

It's all clarifying.

I really do love myself.

I know that I can do a great job in whatever I choose to do."

Let's go to the **Top of Head** now and tap.

"I want you to feel gratitude, gratitude that you have the assertiveness now to ask for what you need. You didn't used to have that. You're becoming clearer in your life about what you want and what you need. And your father is not there intimidating you right now like he used to. You do have the technology now to stay in connection with your mom wherever she is. You're getting old enough that you've got a few more years of school and then you'll get to choose a career. You'll get to choose if sometimes you meet your mother in exotic places and travel with her. You have tools and tapping buddies that can help you to just continue to take off all the layers so that you're just a totally clear channel to create any life of your desire. Just be grateful that you're only 23 years old and you can clear all this stuff now instead of waiting till you've lived with it your whole life.

I love myself.

I love my body.

My body has been trying to send me messages my whole life.

I just didn't have the manual, so I didn't know what the messages meant.

Now I'm starting to understand the body's language.

I'll get better and better.

My body is my temple. Together we are creating a wonderful life together.

I love that.

And so it is."

After this tapping sequence Helen reported: "I feel interesting. At the start of the session I could feel I was wheezing a bit. Now I feel like I can breathe easier. It's not as difficult to breathe in and out. I feel a lot lighter in myself as well."

Appendix 1 –

Multiple Chemical Sensitivity Syndrome

"**Multiple chemical sensitivity (MCS)** is a chronic medical condition characterized by symptoms that the affected person attributes to low-level chemical exposure. Commonly accused substances include smoke, pesticides, plastics, synthetic fabrics, scented products, petroleum products, and paint fumes. Symptoms are often vague and non-specific, such as nausea, fatigue, dizziness and headaches, but also commonly include inflammation of skin, joints, gastrointestinal tract and airways.

MCS is a disputed diagnosis and is controversially not recognized as an organic, chemical-caused illness by the American Medical Association and some other US based organizations. Blinded clinical trials have shown MCS patients react as often and as strongly to placebos, including clean air, as they do to the chemicals they say harm them. This has led some in the healthcare profession to believe MCS symptoms are due to odor hypersensitivity or are mainly psychological.[79] Regardless of the etiology, some people with severe symptoms are disabled as a result.

MCS has been given many different names by proponents, including toxic injury (TI), chemical sensitivity (CS), chemical injury syndrome (CI), 20th century syndrome, environmental illness (EI), sick building syndrome, idiopathic environmental intolerance (IEI), and toxicant-induced loss of tolerance (TILT). These names generally are intended to name the cause favored by the proponent or to emphasize the severity of symptoms."[80]

---

[79] Because this condition is considered to be "mainly psychological", Energy Psychology interventions can be quite effective in resolving the causes on a variety of levels, and after deeply embedded emotional patterns of cause are cleared, other disciplines such as naturopathy can support the faster healing and de-toxing of the body.

[80] To read more go to:
http://en.wikipedia.org/wiki/Multiple_chemical_sensitivity

Appendix 2 –

Pre-coaching Intake Form Questions

Prior to working with each client I send a set of questions to provide the history and clues that I need to best help that client and to save talking time in the first session. My practice is as an energy psychologist, and I choose to spend time in each session clearing energy rather than hearing the "story", so this helps greatly.

- In your own words, what is your main priority issue or condition for scheduling a session?

- If any, what resistance, emotional charge, or challenge do you feel around the above? (ie: Fear? Stress? Frustration? I doubt I can do it? Embarrassed to talk about it? Etc.) - Describe:

- Rate the emotional charge you feel about your priority issue [0=none/neutral- 5=medium charge- 10=highly stressed]

- List all of the specific Emotional Issues or Physical Symptoms you are experiencing right now.

- Now rate each issue on the above list by emotional charge or physical discomfort using the 0-10 scale listed above.

- Provide a list of all medications or homeopathic remedies you are presently taking... and add what condition each is treating.

- Describe your present diet: (non-gluten, paleo, OG/ non-GMO, vegetarian, vegan, traditional southern, etc.)

- List here anything you know about the following from the time of your conception through age 7: (Parent's attitudes about pregnancy with you, mother's pregnancy experience, traumas during pregnancy, early living environment & setting, socio-economic issues, temperaments of parents, over-all tone of your early life, repeated actions, comments, complaints, declarations by others around you, etc.)

- It will be helpful in our work if you list all accidents, physical issues/illnesses, negative emotional life-impacting episodes, surgeries, etc. that have impacted your mind, body, spirit. (You don't need to go into great detail... just list your age and then: "car accident", "divorce", "disappointment", "miscarriage", "job lay-off or lost contract", etc.)

- Threats or Challenges that you are facing now in your life - (What's holding you back?):

- Opportunities, insights, and breakthroughs available to you now – (What is supporting you?):

- What is your main intention for the results of our first session together?

- To provide more information about your body's energetics, please go to http://wellnesscheckonline.com . Then...
- Fill in the questions listing frequency of feelings & symptoms. (Remember that your body & mind are intricately connected, so the data will guide me as to how to support your body-mind-spirit system wholistically.)
- Submit and you will receive the results automatically.
- Print out the two results pages and have available during your first session.
- Use the "Send Results to Practitioner" option and forward to info@arielagroup.com prior to our first session.

Appendix 3 -

Polyvagal Theory

"The Polyvagal Theory introduces a new perspective relating autonomic function to behavior that includes an appreciation of the autonomic nervous system as a "system," the identification of neural circuits involved in the regulation of autonomic state, and an interpretation of autonomic reactivity as adaptive within the context of the phylogeny of the vertebrate autonomic nervous system.[81] The polyvagal perspective explores new questions, paradigms, explanations, and conclusions regarding the role that autonomic function has in the regulation of affective states and social behavior. Foremost, the polyvagal perspective emphasizes the importance of phylogenetic changes in the neural structures regulating the heart and how these phylogenetic shifts provide insights into the adaptive function of both physiology and behavior. The theory emphasizes the phylogenetic emergence of two vagal systems: a potentially lethal ancient circuit involved in defensive strategies of immobilization (e.g., fainting, dissociative states) and a newer mammalian circuit linking the heart to the face that is involved in both social engagement behaviors and in dampening reactivity of the sympathetic nervous system and the Hypothalamic-pituitary-adrenal axis.

The Polyvagal Theory provides a new conceptualization of the autonomic nervous system that emphasizes how an understanding of neurophysiological mechanisms and phylogenetic shifts in the neural regulation of the heart leads to insights into causes and treatments of mental and physical illness.[82] The Polyvagal Theory provides a plausible explanation of several features that are compromised during stress and observed in several psychiatric disorders."[83]

"Summing up just a few of the basics of the polyvagal theory,

---

[81] Porges, S.W. (2003). "The Polyvagal Theory: phylogenetic contributions to social behavior." **Physiology and Behavior**, 79, 503-513.
[82] Porges, S.W. (2007). "The Polyvagal Perspective." **Biological Psychology**, 74, 116-143
[83] **Wikipedia.** (2015) https://en.wikipedia.org/wiki/Stephen_Porges

Porges bases his analysis on an in-depth study of the evolution of the nervous system from the simplest invertebrates to mammalian life and humans in particular. This approach brings with it some important insights. For one, our nervous system is constantly assessing the environment, whether it is safe or not. This process happens without our conscious awareness. Ordinarily, if the environment is safe, we predominantly use our newest "hardware", so to speak. We are socially engaging, communicative. We share, love, nurture, support, play. This is intimately tied with the myelinated vagus, which as a result of evolutionary processes, is intimately tied with heart rate, breathing, and the use of the muscles in the neck, head, and face. All of these are integral to the expression of emotion. But when we encounter a dangerous situation, we revert to an evolutionary 'older' system. We stop engaging socially and instead fight or flee. And if the danger looks hopeless, the primitive vagus takes over, immobilizing us for a painless death. Trauma can leave us stuck in one of those lower circuits, as can various forms of mental illness (autism, PTSD, borderline personality disorder, etc.)."[84]

---

[84] Porges, Stephen W., PhD. (2011) **The Polyvagal Theory: Neurophysiological Foundations of Emotions, Attachment, Communication, and Self-regulation** (Norton Series on Interpersonal Neurobiology). New York: NY/ Norton & Co., Inc. – Amazon book review by Harrison Koehli, July 31, 2011.

Appendix 4 –

Kristen's Leg Photos

This is how Kristen looked when she first presented to me to use Energy Psychology in her healing:

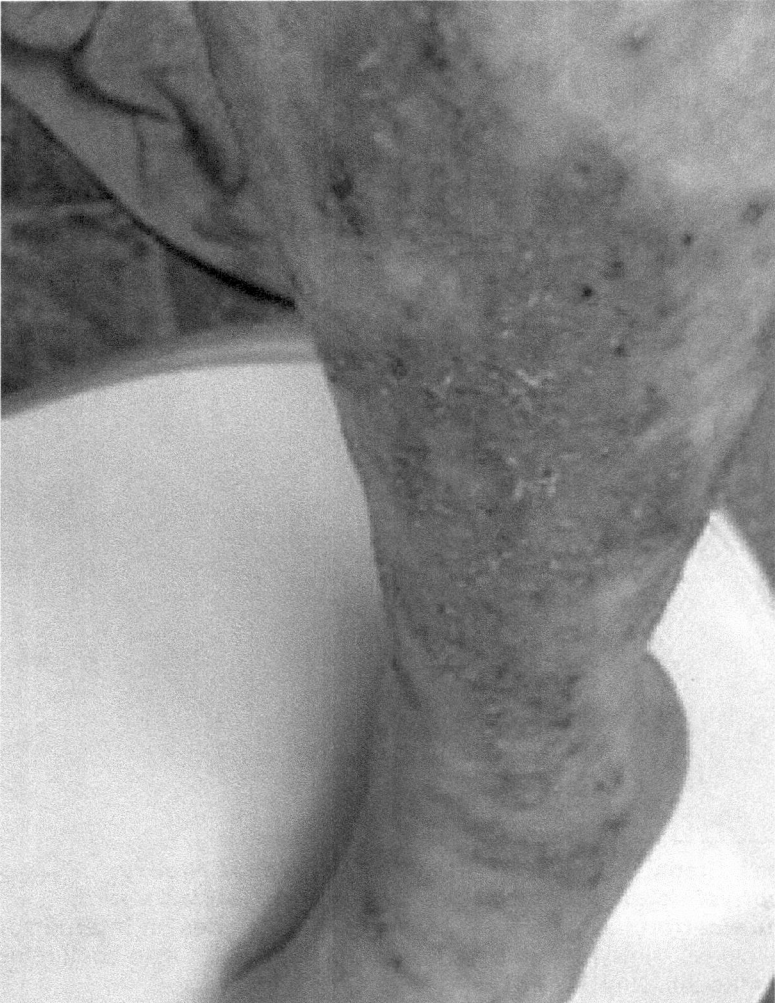

Just one month later the following photo was taken, after we worked on clearing the multiple traumas around:

1. The trauma and loss of losing her father – her favorite parent,
2. Sibling issues: Oldest brother traumas, Oldest sister abusive traumas, Favorite sister's death and loss.
3. Traumatic time at home after her father's death – triggered by her son's family dynamics
4. Fears: about being alone against the IRS, battling her health issues, questions about her future, fears of getting old without enough money to support herself.

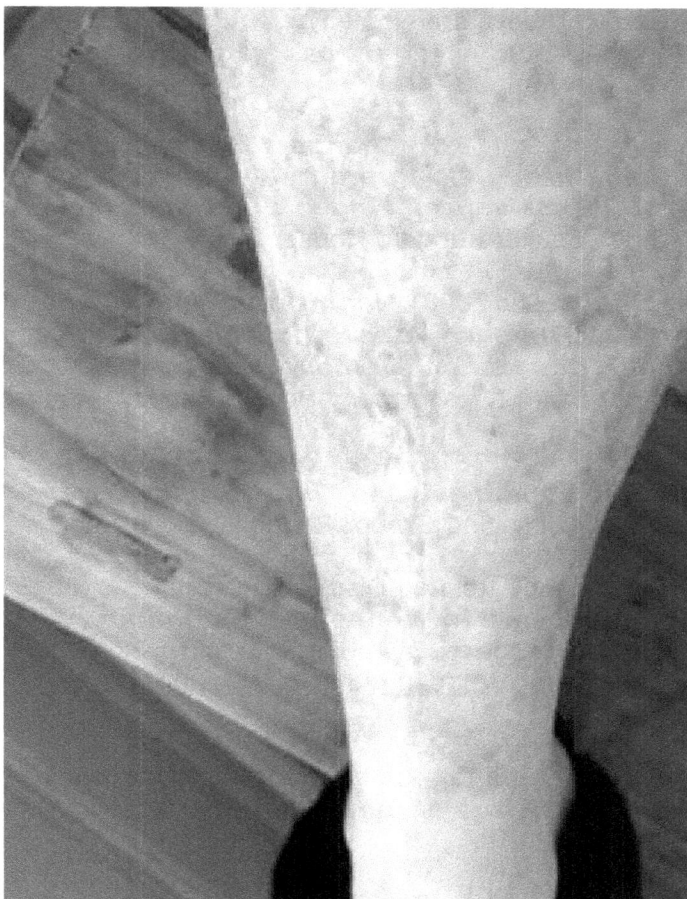

Bibliography of Related Topics

The sources listed below give extensive background for what I have presented in this book as well as for what I shared during my live presentations at the **ACEP/ *Association for Comprehensive Energy Psychology*,** (May 2015), and **ANMA/ *American Naturopathic Medical Association*,** (August 2015), **Annual Conferences**. The data supports basic information for any practitioner wishing to work with the autoimmune audience. While some of these sources refer to the mind-emotion / body connection, others focus on other potential causes of or attributing factors in autoimmune. It is my hypothesis that all suggested "scientifically proven causes" correlate dramatically with underlying emotional factors... and that natural interventions are proving very effective in leading to rebalancing and cure.

Amen, Daniel G., M.D. (1998) *Change Your brain Change Your Life: The Breakthrough Program for Conquering Anxiety, Depression, Obsessiveness, Anger, and Impulsiveness.* New York, NY: Times Books/ Random House, Inc.

Amen, Daniel G., M.D. (2008) *Magnificent Mind at Any Age: Natural Ways to Unleash Your Brain's Maximum Potential – Treat Anxiety, Depression, Memory Problems, ADD, and Insomnia.* New York, NY: Harmony Books/ Random House, Inc.

Amen, Daniel G., M.D. (2012) *Use Your Brain to Change Your Age: Secrets to Look, Feel, and Think Younger Every Day.* New York, NY: Crown Publishing Group/ Random House, Inc.

American Autoimmune Related Diseases Association. (2015) **"Autoimmune Disease in Women; Autoimmunity: A Major Women's Health Issue"**. Eastpointe, MI: http://aarda.org https://www.aarda.org/autoimmune-information/autoimmune-disease-in-women

Anderson, Warwick, and Ian R. Mackay. (2014) *Intolerant Bodies: A Short History of Autoimmunity.* Baltimore, MD: John Hopkins University Press.

Ballantyne, S., PhD. (2013) *The Paleo Approach: Reverse

Autoimmune Disease and Heal Your Body. USA: Victory Belt Publishing.

Blome, Gotz, MD. (1992) *Advanced Bach Flower Therapy: A Scientific Approach to Diagnosis and Treatment*. Rochester, Vermont: Healing Arts Press.

Blum, S., MD, MPH with Bender, M. (2013) *The Immune System Recovery Plan: A Doctor's 4-Step Program to Treat Autoimmune Disease.* New York, NY: Scribner Publishing.

Castro, Miranda, FSHom. (1997) *Homeopathic Guide to Stress: Safe and Effective Natural Ways to Alleviate Physical and Emotional Stress.* New York, NY: St. Martin's Griffin.

Challem, Jack. (2010) *The Inflammation Syndrome: Your Nutrition Plan for Great Health, Weight Loss, and Pain-Free Living.* Hoboken, NJ: John Wiley & Sons, Inc.

Chappell, Peter, FSHom. (1994) *Emotional Healing with Homeopathy: A Self Help Manual*. Rockport, MA: Element Publishers.

Chopra, Deepak, M.D. & Tanzi, Rudolf E., Ph.D. (2012) *Super Brain: Unleashing the Explosive Power of Your Mind to Maximize Health, Happiness, and Spiritual Well-Being*. NY, NY: Harmony Books.

Church, Dawson, PhD. (2007) *The Genie in Your Genes: Epigenetic Medicine and the New Biology of Intention.* Santa Rosa, CA: Elite Books.

Crook, William G., MD. (1986) *The Yeast Connection – A Medical Breakthrough: If You Feel Sick All Over, This Book Could Change Your Life*. Jackson, TN: Professional Books.

Edelson, S. B., MD & Mitchell, D. (2003). *What Your Doctor May Not Tell You About Autoimmune Disorders; The Revolutionary Drug-free Treatments for Thyroid Disease, Lupus, MS, IBD, Chronic Fatigue, Rheumatoid Arthritis, and Other Diseases*. New York, NY: Warner Books, Inc.

Eden, Donna, with Feinstein, D., PhD (2008) *Energy Medicine: Balancing Your Body's Energies for Optimal Health, Joy, and Vitality.* New York, NY: Penguin Group Publishers.

EFT & Beyond: Cutting Edge Techniques for Personal Transformation. (2009) Bruner, Pamela & Bullough, John, Editors. Saffron Waldon, UK: Energy Publications Ltd.

Feinstein, David, PhD; Eden, Donna; & Craig, Gary. (2005) *The Promise of Energy Psychology: Revolutionary Tools for Dramatic Personal Change.* New York, NY: Tarcher/Penguin.

Fife, Bruce, C.N., N.D. (2004) *The Coconut Oil Miracle: Use nature's elixir to: lose weight -prevent heart disease, cancer, diabetes – strengthen the immune system – beautify skin and hair.* New York, NY: Avery/ Penguin Group, Inc.

Frost, R. (2002*) Applied Kinesiology: A Training Manual and Reference Book of Basic Principles and Practices.* Berkeley, CA: North Atlantic Books.

Fuhrman, Joel, M.D. (2013) *The Eat to Live Plan to Prevent and Reverse Diabetes.* NY, NY: Harper One/ Harper Collins Publishers.

Gittleman, Ann Louise. (2014) *Zapped: Why Your Cell Phone Shouldn't Be Your Alarm Clock and 1,268 Ways to Outsmart the Hazards of Electronic Pollution.* New York, NY: Harper Collins Publishers.

Goldstein, Cathy, A.P.; Dterman, Kevin, D.C. (2010) **"The Body Can Not Heal If the Lymphatics are Plugged"**, *The 2010 NET Seminars EAGLES Presentations*. Carlsbad, CA: N.E.T. Inc. www.NETmindbody.com

Graham, Linda. (2013) *Bouncing Back: Rewiring Your Brain for Maximum Resilience and Well-Being.* Novato, CA: New World Library.

Green, Debra. (2010) www.RadiationPage.com **"Electromagnetic Frequencies (EMF) and Your Health"** via http://YourEnergyMatters.com .

Haas, Rue. (2012) "Fibromyalgia: An Energy Imbalance" – **The Tapping Solution website.** August 3, 2012. http://www.thetappingsolution.com/eft-articles/fibromyalgia-an-energy-imbalance [Her mention of the location of the spleen point is incorrect... the protocol is good for the chin point Central meridian, and including the under arm Spleen meridian is also potent for her intentions.]

Hay, Louise. (1984) *Heal Your Body.* Carlsbad, CA: Hay House.

Junger, A., MD (2013) *Clean Gut: The Breakthrough Plan for Eliminating the Root Cause of Disease and Revolutionizing Your Health.* New York, NY: HarperCollins Publishers, Inc.

Junger, Alejandro, M.D. with Amely Greeven. (2009) *Clean: The Revolutionary Program to Restore the Body's Natural Ability to Heal Itself.* New York, NY: Harper Collins.

Korn, Danna. (2010) *Living Gluten-Free for Dummies*. 2nd Edition. Hoboken, NJ: John Wiley & Sons Publishers.

Kudlas, Michael, D.C., M.A., M.Ed. (1998) **"Levels of Consciousness & Working Before Conception Some Precautions"**, *NET Gathering of the Eagles – 10th Anniversary*. Encinitas, CA: N.E.T., Inc.

Lahita, R.G., MD, PhD with Yalof I. (2004). *Women & Autoimmune Disease: The Mysterious Ways Your Body Betrays Itself.* New York, NY: HarperCollins Publishers, Inc.

Leary, Mark, Ph.D. (2012). *Understanding the Mysteries of Human Behavior*: **Course Guidebook & Audio.** Chantilly, VA: The Great Courses Publishers.

Lepore, D., ND. (1985). *The Ultimate Healing System: The Illustrated Guide to Muscle Testing & Nutrition.* New Jersey: Woodland Publishing, Inc.

Lipton, Bruce H., Ph.D. (2008) 2nd Edition. *The Biology of Belief:*

Unleashing the Power of Consciousness, Matter & Miracles.
Hay House Publishers: www.hayhouse.com

Mate', Gabor, MD. (2011) *When the Body Says No: The Cost of Hidden Stress – Exploring the Stress-Disease Connection*.
Hoboken, NJ: John Wiley & Sons.

MedlinePlus. *(2015)* **"Autoimmune Diseases",** *MedlinePlus: Trusted Health Information for You*.
http://www.nlm.nih.gov/medlineplus/autoimmunediseases.html

Meinig, G.E., DDS, FACD (2008) *Root Canal Cover-Up: A Founder of the Association of Root Canal Specialists Discovers Evidence That Root Canals Damage Your Health – Learn What to Do.* La Mesa, CA: Price-Pottenger Nutrition Foundation.

Merkel, Anne, Ph.D. (2015) *Autoimmune Cases – Naturally! Treating Autoimmune Disorders Using Energy Psychology and Naturopathy.* Mineral Bluff, GA: Ariela Group Publications.
http://is.gd/AnnesBooks

Merkel, Anne, Ph.D. (2014) "Classic EFT Set-Up Statement May Benefit Autoimmune Cases" – **The Tapping Solution Website.**
March 26, 2014. http://www.thetappingsolution.com/eft-articles/classic-eft-set-up-statement-may-help-autoimmune-cases

Merkel, Anne, Ph.D. (2014) "Clearing Early Abuse Issues Causing Autoimmune Disorders " – **The Tapping Solution Website.** March 26, 2014. http://www.thetappingsolution.com/eft-articles/clearing-early-abuse-issues-causing-autoimmune-disorders

Merkel, Anne, Ph.D. (2015) *Conscious Development Guide for EFT Tapping Practitioners.* Mineral Bluff, GA: Ariela Group Publications. http://is.gd/AnnesBooks

Merkel, Anne, Ph.D. (2015) *EFT–Best Practices for Energy Management.* Mineral Bluff, GA: Ariela Group Publications.
http://is.gd/AnnesBooks

Merkel, Anne, Ph.D. (2013) "Issues Underlying Autoimmune Disorders" – **The Tapping Solution Website**. Sept. 12, 2013.

http://www.thetappingsolution.com/eft-articles/issues-underlying-autoimmune-disorders

Merkel, Anne, Ph.D. (2015) "Tapping for 'Surface Pain' of Autoimmune Disorders " – **The Tapping Solution Website.** May 11, 2015. http://www.thetappingsolution.com/eft-articles/tapping-for-surface-pain-of-autoimmune-disorders

Merkel, Anne, Ph.D. (2013) "Tapping the 'Heart Center' for Autoimmune Disorders " – **The Tapping Solution Website.** Sept. 16, 2013. http://www.thetappingsolution.com/eft-articles/tapping-the-heart-center-for-autoimmune-disorders

Merkel, Anne, Ph.D. (2015) *Transformative Coaching Guidebook for EFT & Energy Therapy Practitioners.* Mineral Bluff, GA: Ariela Group Publications. http://is.gd/AnnesBooks

Nelson, Bradley, D.C. (2007) *The Emotion Code: How to Release Your Trapped Emotions for Abundant Health, Love, and Happiness.* Mesquite, NV: Wellness Unmasked Publishing.

Ober, Clinton; Sinatra, Stephen T., M.D.; Zucker, Martin. (2010) *Earthing: The most important health discovery ever?* Laguna Beach, CA:; Basic Health Publications, Inc. www.basichealthpub.com

Oelke, Jane, N.D., Ph.D. (2001) *Natural Choices for Fibromyalgia: Discover Your Personal method for Pain Relief.* Stevensville, MI: Natural Choices, Inc. www.NaturalChoicesForYou.com

Ortner, Nick. (2013) *The Tapping Solution: A Revolutionary System for Stress-Free Living.* Carlsbad, CA: Hay House, Inc.

Oschman, James L., PhD. (2000) *Energy Medicine: The Scientific Basis.* New York, NY: Churchill Livingstone.

Panos, Maesimund B., MD, and Jane Heimlich. (1980) *Homeopathic Medicine at Home: Natural Remedies for Everyday Ailments and Minor Injuries.* New York, NY: Tarcher/Putnam Publishers of Penguin Putnam, Inc.

Pease, Roger W., Jr., Editor. (2006) **Merriam-Webster's Medical Dictionary.** Springfield, MA: Merriam-Webster, Inc.

Pert, Candace B., Ph.D. (1997) **Molecules of Emotion: The Science Behind Mind-Body Medicine.** New York, NY: Scribner.

Porges, S.W. (2007). "The Polyvagal Perspective." **Biological Psychology**, 74, 116-143.

Porges, Stephen W., PhD. (2011) **The Polyvagal Theory: Neurophysiological Foundations of Emotions, Attachment, Communication, and Self-regulation** (Norton Series on Interpersonal Neurobiology). New York: NY/ Norton & Co., Inc.

Porges, S.W. (2003). "The Polyvagal Theory: phylogenetic contributions to social   behavior." **Physiology and Behavior**, 79, 503-513.

Ryce, Michael, ND. (1997) **Why is This Happening to Me... Again?!... and What You Can Do About It!** Theodosia, Missouri: dr. michael ryce, whyagain@kcmo.com .

Shames, R., MD & Shames, K., PhD, RN & Shames, G.G., LAc (2011) **Thyroid Mind Power: The Proven Cure for Hormone-Related Depression, Anxiety, and Memory Loss.** New York, NY: Rodale, Inc.

Shealy, C. Norman, MD, PhD. (2011) **Energy Medicine: Practical Applications and Scientific Proof.** Virginia Beach, VA: ARE Press.

Shomon, M. J. (2002**). Living Well With Autoimmune Disease: What Your Doctor Doesn't Tell You... That You Need To Know.** New York, NY: HarperCollins Publishers, Inc.

Sodi, Carla M. (2015) "PART 1: The Bond Between Autoimmune Diseases and Highly Sensitive Persons". April 13, 2015. "PART 2: The Hidden Link Between Highly Sensitive People and Autoimmune Disorders" –**The Tapping Solution Website**
   http://www.thetappingsolution.com/eft-articles/category/carla-m-sodi

Taylor, Jill Bolte, Ph.D. (2006) *My Stroke of Insight: A Brain Scientist's Personal Journey.* New York, NY: Viking Press.

Thie, John, DC, and Matthew Thie, M.Ed. (2007) *Touch for Health – A Practical Guide to Natural Health with Acupressure Touch.* The Complete Edition. Camarillo, CA: DeVorss Publications. http://www.touchforhealth.us/

Toney, T. (2010). *Get Clean Go Green EcoDiet: The Secrets of an Alkaline Environment.* USA: New Earth Publishers.

Van Der Kolk, Bessel. (2014) *The Body Keeps the Score: Brain, Mind, & Body in the Healing of Trauma.* New York, NY: Viking Penguin Group.

Velasquez-Manoff, Moises. (2012) *An Epidemic of Absence: A New Way of Understanding Allergies and Autoimmune Diseases.* New York, NY: Scribner.

Wahls, T., MD (2014). *The Wahls Protocol: How I Beat Progressive MS Using Paleo Principles and Functional Medicine.* New York, NY: Penguin Group Publishers.

Walker, Scott, D.C. (1994) *NET Remedies Practitioner's Support Manual.* Encinitas, CA: N.E.T., Inc. www.NETmindbody.com

Walker, Scott, D.C. (1996) *NET Results: An Established Format for Those Difficult Cases Which Need In-depth Care.* Encinitas, CA: N.E.T., Inc. www.NETmindbody.com

Wauters, Ambika. (2007) *The Homeopathy Bible.* New York, NY: Sterling Publishing, Inc.

Wilson, J.L., ND, DC, PhD. (2011) *Adrenal Fatigue: The 21st Century Stress Syndrome – What it is and how you can recover.* Petaluma, CA: Smart Publications.

About the Author

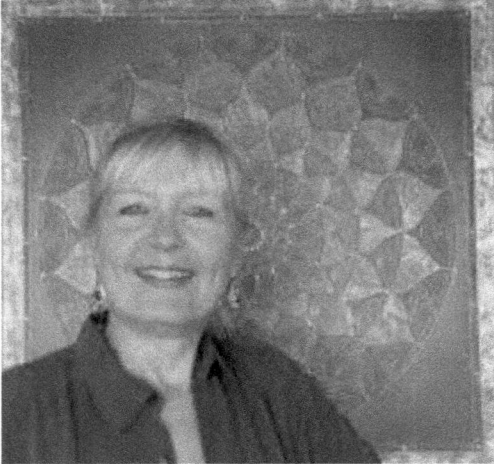

Anne Merkel, PhD, CNHP, has researched and implemented cognitive, cultural, energetic, psychological, and physical techniques and interventions for over forty years.

Her practice as an Energy Psychologist with those suffering from autoimmune disorders pulls together her extensive work in Energy Therapies, Naturopathy, and Energy Medicine, sharing techniques used across a variety of functional medicine disciplines.

Dr. Merkel trains and certifies licensed Health and Wellness Practitioners of all kinds as well as EFT Tapping Practitioners. Her research points out how beneficial it is to other health interventions if the emotional stress is cleared before the intervention is administered. Many Functional Medicine Practitioners are incorporating Energy Therapy and Energy Psychology into their practices with noticeable results. It has become clear that for true "healing" to occur the body-mind-spirit system must be approached in a whole sense so that all parts can re-balance in the ways nature intended.

For more information about Dr. Anne Merkel and her practice, programs, publications, and research you may go to:

http://AnneMerkel.com

http://ArielaGroup.com

http://MyEFTCoach.com

http://AlchemistAnne.com

http://is.gd/AnnesBooks

www.ingramcontent.com/pod-product-compliance
Lightning Source LLC
Chambersburg PA
CBHW072125270326
41931CB00010B/1671